DIGITAL PHOTOGRAPHY IN ORTHODONTICS

A Practical Guide For Clinical Excellence

Niharika Goyal

MDS (Orthodontics and Dentofacial Orthopaedics)

Presently at, Akash Hospital, Samalkha, Harayana, India

Tanika Gupta

MDS (Orthodontics and Dentofacial Orthopaedics)

Presently Senior lecturer, IDS, Sehora, Jammu, India

Made with ♥ on the Notion Press Platform
www.notionpress.com

DEDICATED TO OUR FAMILY

PREFACE

High-quality clinical photography is essential in orthodontics, playing a crucial role in diagnosis, treatment planning, patient education and professional communication. However, capturing consistently clear and detailed orthodontic photographs can be challenging, particularly without knowledge of standardized techniques and equipment. Using easily recognised facial landmarks, dental photographs can standardise frontal and lateral portraits for more consistent comparison, and by standardisation they could become valuable additions to clinical charts/records. So, this book provides a comprehensive guide on the key elements of effective orthodontic photography, including camera settings, positioning and lighting. Illustrating each step in the process that aims to equip orthodontists with skills needed to achieve high-quality, reproducible clinical photos that enhance the quality of patient care and support clinical documentation.

CONTENTS

INTRODUCTION

Modern dentistry, as a part of the complete therapy plan, includes the whole of the patient's face. A photograph provides important visual reference for monitoring growth and developmental changes, providing the patient with a view of the changes and providing the therapist with credible visual material for teaching and research. The first component to consider is the technical aspect of photography.

Photography in dentistry has made some change and progress since ***Nov 1968***. Photographic information for the health professional has little or no standard.

The word photograph comes from Greek Work ***(phos-light, Graphein – to draw)meaning to write or draw with light***. A photograph is basically a picture drawn with rays of light.

However, documentation of the treatment with pre-treatment and post-treatment photographs can be misleading if the features on one or both photographs are distorted. Clinical photographs allow the orthodontist to carefully study the existing patient'ssoft-tissue patterns during the treatment planning stage.

Consequently, numerous frontal and lateral photographs are taken with different head and camera positions in order to show their different contributions to the final picture. Using easily recognised facial landmarks, dental photographers can standardise frontal and lateral portraits for more consistent comparison, and by standardisation they could become valuable additions to clinical charts/records.

At some time in our lives we have all used a camera, but clinical dental photography doesn't lend itself well to the concept of "point and shoot".

The nature of the environment, the small sizes and distances involved, and the difficulty of access make dental photography an art as well as a science. And like science, there are rules that have to be obeyed, such as focus, exposure and composition. But as with art, results improve with practice and experience.

The majority of dentofacial changes are usually monitored by the method of cephalometry, where the structures of soft tissues are only registered in profile, and anteroposterior presentation is made impossible. As patients do not understand their own cephalogram, and neither do they know how to interpret the cephalometric analysis, the photograph represents a much more conventional documentation of the soft tissues and also a visual reference for monitoring the changes which occur during growth and development.

It is a reliable source for qualitative evaluation of postoperative results, as the patient is enabled a review of his own changes prior to and after certain operations, and the therapist can use it as visual material in teaching or as the basis for further research. There is an increasing need for such photo-documentation in orthodontics, as in many other dental disciplines.

As an adjunct to the practice of dentistry, clinical photography brings rewards such as a sense of satisfaction in a job well done, the ability to share one's work with colleagues and patients, and a great opportunity to advance your dental practice.

Orthodontic records have always been very important in Orthodontics since they are a basic diagnostic tool which tells us about the patient occlusion. This information will be very useful to make and plan a right diagnosis and orthodontic treatment.

Basic orthodontic records include three main types of records:

Study Models	Properly-trimmed, stone-cast moulds of the dentition.
Radiographs	Normally a panorax (OPG) and a Lateral Cephalometric Vie
Clinical photographs	Pre treatment and post treatment , intraoral and extra

	oral photographs.

It is becoming increasingly important that high quality clinical records are taken as part of a course of orthodontic treatment. Study models tend to be the one record that is consistently taken for orthodontic patients throughout the world. The quality of study models is very variable and unless great care is taken both with the impressions themselves, with the wax registration bite, and with the choice of laboratory, study models can end up offering less clinical information than is ideally required. Clinical photographs, however, can offer at least as much, if not more, information provided care is taken when obtaining these photographs.

Currently the intra oral color photography is included by the orthodontists among their case records pretreatment, post treatment, and possibly post retention. ***These photographs complement the other orthodontic records – study casts, intra oral and extra oral radiographs and facial photographs.***

Colored photographs play a very important clinical and legal role. They record the status of the oral soft and hard tissue, especially pretreatment oral hygiene status, gingival health, and the presence of enamel defects, both congenital and acquired.

From a diagnostic point of view, what might not make a mental imprint on intra oral examination will make a strong impression when a slide is projected onto a screen and enlarged.

Intra oral photographs also provide a valuable aid in case presentations, as they are visually more striking to parents and patients than white plaster casts. In fact, a series of photographic slides documenting the progress of treatment in certain types of cases is an excellent visual aid.

Case presentations to study clubs and other groups would be greatly improved if, in addition to pre-and post-treatment slides, serial photographs taken throughout the treatment period to document treatment mechanics were also shown. Many orthodontists already do this in selected cases, but it is time consuming and the photographic results are not always entirely satisfactory.

Excellent documentation systems, including medical and dental histories, complete clinical examinations, diagnosis and treatment plan protocols, and juries in determining whether the doctor provided proper patient care carefully consider thorough informed consent. Also, it is important to provide extensive informed consent, especially when proceeding with the alternative treatment plan. If there is one word to remember, proper documentation will be the only unbiased testimony presented at trial. Either party may attempt to clear their testimony, but the unaltered office records, treatment chart, and correspondence will speak louder and clearer and will confirm what the doctor states in the deposition and at the trial with thorough informed consent practices, patients will be aware of the options they have and can then make intelligent decisions for which they will assume responsibility. In the long run, both the patient and the orthodontist will benefit from these procedures.

BASIC PHOTOGRAPHY

What is Photography?

The complete process by which pictures are made by the chemical action of light on a sensitized plate or film is known as photography. Many chemicals are sensitive to and affected by light. *A common example is: salt of silver chloride darkens by prolonged exposure to light.*

To make a picture, first of all a chemically prepared surface is needed, which is generally a uniform coating over glass, celluloid or paper. An emulsion of insoluble silver halides and gelatin is prepared and then its coating is done on glass, celluloid or paper. All this has to be done in total darkness.

The camera is a wonderful little instrument for producing pictures. It is a ***light-tight box with a lens fitted in the front.*** There is an arrangement for keeping the sensitive surface i.e. plate or film at the back. For the light to reach the film, through the lens, there is a device known as the shutter. The purpose of the lens is to form an image of the object at the back within the camera, where the film is kept. The formed image is real but inverted. When the shutter is released for some small and appropriate duration of time, an exposure is said to have been given to the film. At this stage, if the film is examined, no image will be visible. However, a latent image would be formed on the emulsion coating on the film. When treated with developer, the film produces an image that is visible.

The process of developing the film and plates is conducted in total darkness. However, in a few cases, a very weak red light can be used.

The developed image will be in black and white. The parts which get more light become darker and those which get less light remain transparent.

The reason is that silver salts are reduced to metallic black silver by the action of the developer and exposure to light.

After developing, the film is kept in the fixer, which dissolves and removes all unexposed silver salts and those areas become transparent. This is the way a negative is prepared, which is just the reverse of the object. To get a correct reproduction of the object the negative is put in contact with photographic paper, which is also coated with an emulsion of silver salts and is exposed to white light through a printing box.

On developing the exposed paper and fixing it, the object appears in its proper order. ***This final result is called a <u>positive</u>***. Bigger and enlarged pictures can also be made from the same negative with the help of an apparatus known as ***<u>Enlarger</u>***.

HISTORY OF PHOTOGRAPHY

Photography was not discovered by any single person. As such, it was the result of constant research in the field of chemistry and physics. As far back in***14th century***, someone happened to go to a darkened room in one of the doors in which there was a very small hole and rays of sunlight passing through this hole, forming a true but inverted image of the outside scene on the opposite wall of the darkened room. In the year ***1569 Della Porta of Italy*** discovered the possibilities of using a glass lens in the place of the hole for a sharp projection of the image of the outside landscape.

As all discoveries go, this was again taken up and in ***1686, Johann Zahn*** described in his Journal the construction of a portable type of instrument with a lens and a mirror to present the image with the right side up (on the same principles as the single lens reflex of today).

At this stage the problem was how to make this image permanent on some sort of surface like paper or glass. In the ***18th century, Gaber*** found out that silver chloride becomes dark when exposed to white light, but nothing further was done in this direction till ***1727, when G.H. Schulze*** made an emulsion of silver nitrate and chalk and coated it on a sheet of metal. Then he placed a transparent paper with some opaque words written on it in contact with the coated metal sheet and exposed it to the sunlight. The coated surface below the words was not exposed and was found white, while the surrounding areas turned black. In the year ***1777, Charles William Scheele*** did some experiments with silver chloride under the influence of various coloured lights. He discovered that red and yellow light had very little effect but other lights completely darkened silver chloride.

In ***1780*** silhouette pictures were made on a paper coated with silver salt solution, by keeping the head of a person in the beam of sunlight and sharp shadows thus created were received on the coated paper. In ***1802 Thomas Wedgwood and Sir Humphrey Davy*** also discovered similar phenomena.

Now the problem was to fix the image on the coated paper and to save it from becoming black on exposure to light. In the late ***18th century, Sir John Herschel*** discovered sodium thyosulphate as a fixing agent.

In the year ***1824*** some pictures on glass and metal sheets were made by ***Joseph Nicephore of France***. He coated the glass with a layer of bitumen dissolved in the oil of lavender and then after treatment with an acid he obtained a negative to produce a positive.

It was not until ***1839 when Mand Daguerre*** prepared a mixture of silver chloride and iodide and coated it on metal plate. Then he gave an exposure for about three hours in the camera but got a very faint image. One day, due to very dull light he kept his exposed plate after removing it from his camera in his chemical cabinet to reuse it. But next day he found that the image on the exposed plate was perfect and clearly visible but he could not understand how it happened. Later he found that it was due to vapors from a bowl of mercury. Thus the first developing agent was discovered by him. He published the details of his method on the request of the French Govt. and named in ***Daguerreotype.***

In ***1841, W.H. Fox Talbot*** prepared for the first time a photography paper for making negatives and positives and named his process as ***Talbotype or Calotype***. In the year ***1849,*** he prepared the glossy type paper also.

In***1851, Scott Archer of London*** introduced his collodion wet plate method of making negatives in the camera. In ***1871 Dr. R.L. Maddox*** invented the present dry plate, using gelatin in place of collodion. In ***1898 Reverend Hannibal Goodwin*** of America introduced the Roll Films which were commercially prepared by Eastman Kodak Company for the first time.

THE CAMERA

For photography, the most essential thing is the camera. All cameras are good and each has its own advantages and disadvantages. When buying a camera one must take into consideration the type of work he or she is going to do. It will depend on the individual taste, choice, and the result one wants to achieve.

- *The term camera is shortened from camera obscura, literally "dark room" in Latin. The camera is basically a box, with small aperture or opening where the lens is attached at one end and the film at the other.*
- *The inside of the camera must be completely dark, so that the rays of light reach the film only through the aperture.*

PRINCIPLE:

- *The camera works in much the same way as the eye.*
- *The lens in the eye focuses the image on to the nerve cells in the retina and this image is sent to the brain by the optic nerve.*

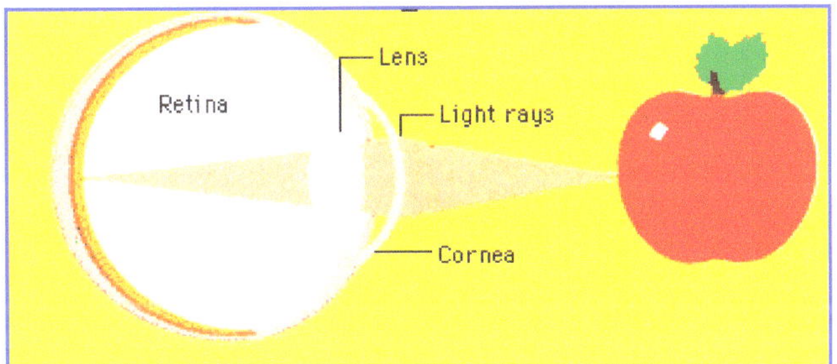

- *This is the principle employed in the camera. The lens sharply focuses the image on to the film.*
- *To keep the image sharp even when the distance varies, the lens has to be moved either farther or closer to the film. This is what is commonly called 'focussing'.*
- *The diaphragm of the camera is a variable aperture, which controls the amount of light allowed onto the film, much in the same way that the iris*

of the human eye contracts in bright sunlight but opens when the room is dark.

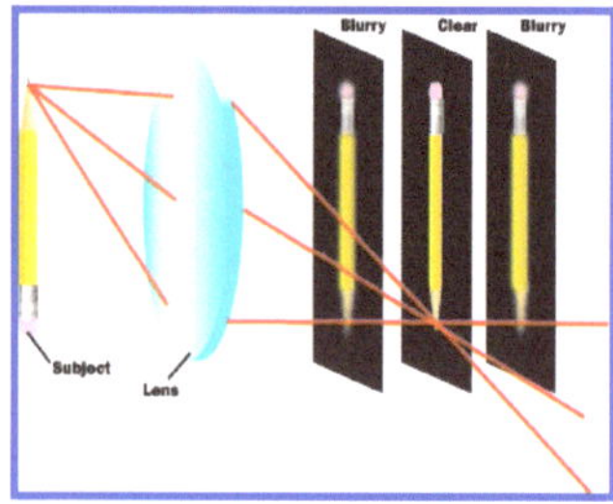

- *The light reflects from a subject, enters the camera through the lens, which focuses the rays of light into an image on the film.*
- *Light rays from the top of the subject form the lower part of the image and those from the bottom form the upper part. Thus, the image on the film is upside down.*

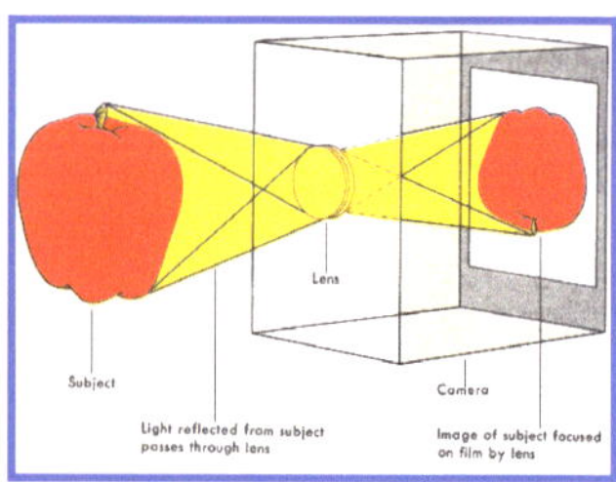

PARTS OF THE CAMERA

1. *Body,*
2. *Lens,*
3. *Shutter and*
4. *View – finder*

1. The body: It is made of die-cast sheet metal or some synthetic material and is light-tight, usually covered with leather or plastic to give a good finish. It is made to open from the back, so that an unexposed film can be fitted into it. There are two chambers in it; one chamber accommodates the new film, the other is for the empty spool. In between these two chambers the film runs behind a metal opening, which frames the picture area. A spring-loaded pressure plate is always fitted inside the back cover of the body, which keeps the film or plate flat and pressed. After one exposure the film is transported to the next frame by a knob or the winding lever on the outside of the body. In a simple box camera, there is a window in the back cover, covered with red plastic, through which the frame number of the film on the backing paper can be seen; but in modern and advanced cameras, frame numbers come automatically, once the film is loaded.

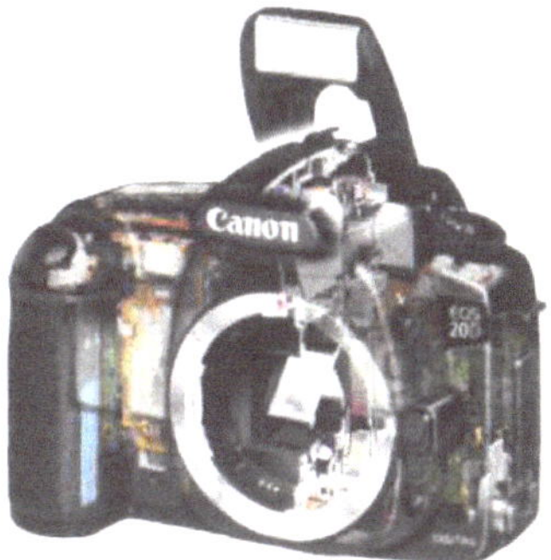

Cross-section of a modern digital single lens reflex camera.

2. The lens:Lens is a piece of transparent material that has at least one curved surface.***The lens is the heart of the camera,*** the component that turns the three dimensional world outside the camera into a two dimensional image on the film inside.Its job is to take the beams of light bouncing off of an object and redirect them so they come together to form a real image -- an image that looks just like the scene in front of the lens.

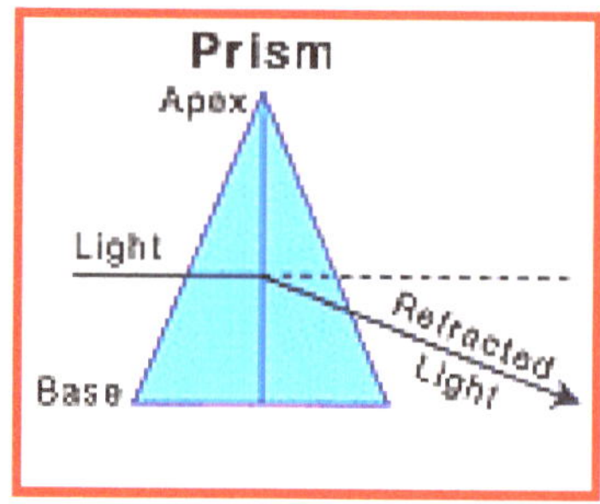

A **lens** can be thought of as two rounded prisms joined together. Light passing through the lens is always bent toward the thickest part of prism.

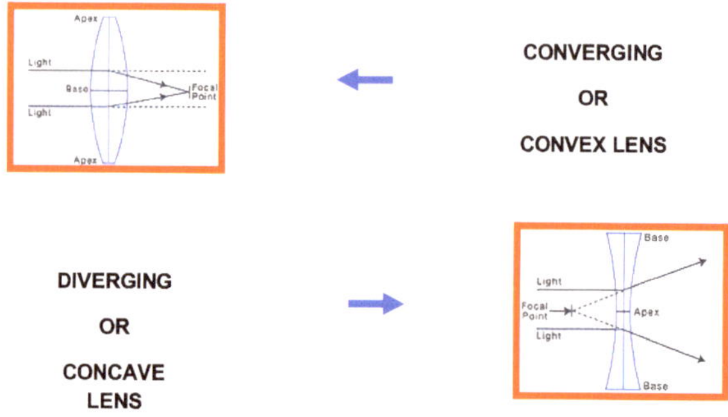

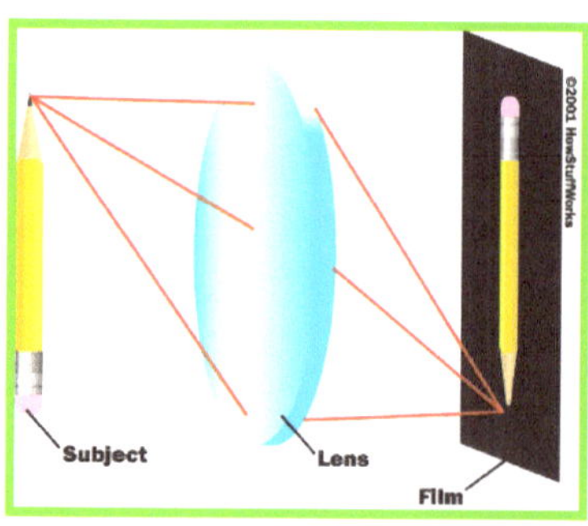

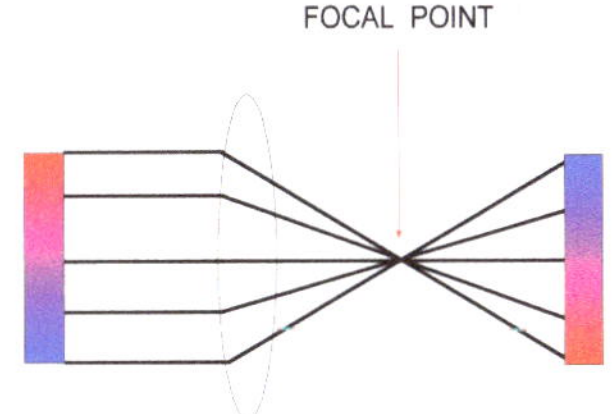

Because of the curvature of the lens surfaces, different rays of an incident light beam are refracted through different angles. Thus, an entire beam of parallel rays can be caused to converge on a single point. This point is called the focal point, or principal focus, of the lens.Refraction of the rays of light reflected from or emitted by an object causes the rays to form a visual image of the object.

This image may be either

- Real-photographable or visible on a screen or
- Virtual-visible only upon looking into the lens, as in a microscope.

The focal length of a lens is the distance from the centre of the lens to the point at which the image of a distant object is formed.

A long-focus lens forms a larger image of a distant object, while a short-focus lens forms a small image.

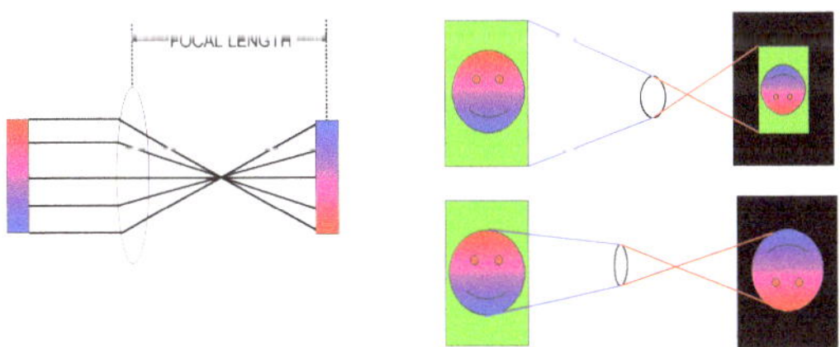

The closer that you move an object to the lens, the larger it will appear on the film or photograph.

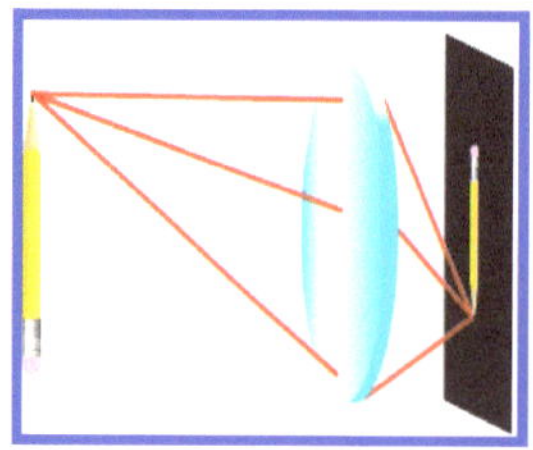

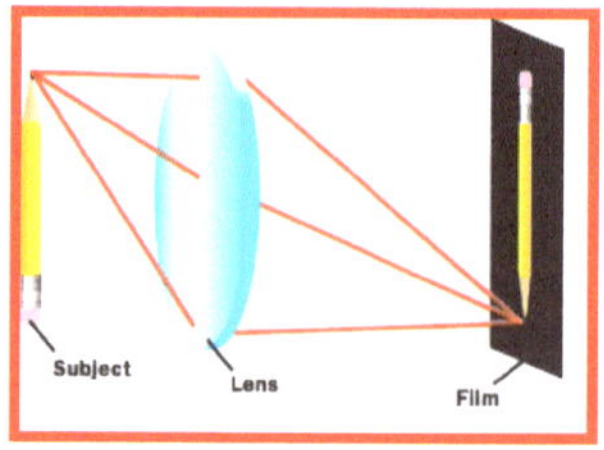

The image may be much larger or smaller than the object, depending on

- the distance between the lens and the object and
- the focal length of the lens

There is a limit to how close you can move an object in order to enlarge an image size. If you move too close to an object, with a lens, which is not suited to that distance, then the image will get distorted. This is one of the most important concepts in dental photography, with regard to lenses.

In an ordinary box and ***instamatic*** type camera the lens is a single piece of glass. This is not optically corrected except in a few cases where a double lens is used. These lenses produce fairly sharp images. In modern and expensive single lens and twin lens reflex and rangefinder type miniature cameras, lenses are ***anastigmatic*** of several components cemented together and these produce very sharp, accurate and undistorted images on the film. These lenses are always coated and show a ***light blue colour***. Such lenses are also capable of reducing internal reflections inside the camera, and thus, image is comparatively clear and sharp, with natural colours or tones.

INTERCHANGEABLE LENSES :(TYPES OF LENSES)

For single lens reflex type camera as a variety of lenses are available in the market like normal, wide angle, telephoto, zoom, macro etc. These lenses are used for photographing different subjects from long to close distance or to cover a large or a small area.

- **Fisheye lenses**: The fish eye is an ultra-wide angled lens. Typically, it will have a focal length of between 6 and 16 m. For shooting interiors or other confined spaces where an extreme angle of view is needed.

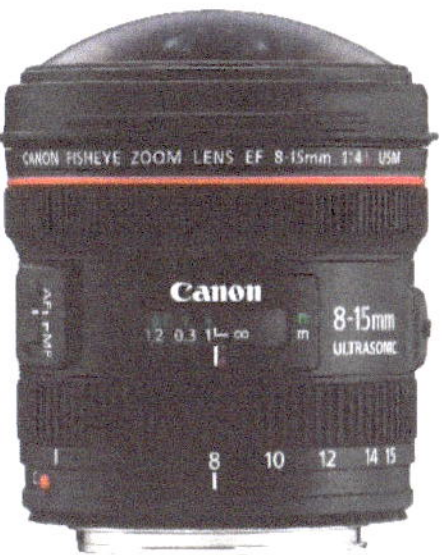

- **Telephoto lens:** When a lens has the focal length greater than the diagonal of the negative, it is known as long focus lens or telephoto lens. This lens has a narrow field of view and has large focal length and show the object larger than what one sees through a normal lens. Thus, objects reproduced in the negatives are much bigger.

Telephoto lenses have a very shallow depth of field and are made in 80 mm to 1,000 mm and some even up to 2,000 mm focal length. These lenses are very useful for pictorial, nature, candid and press photography.

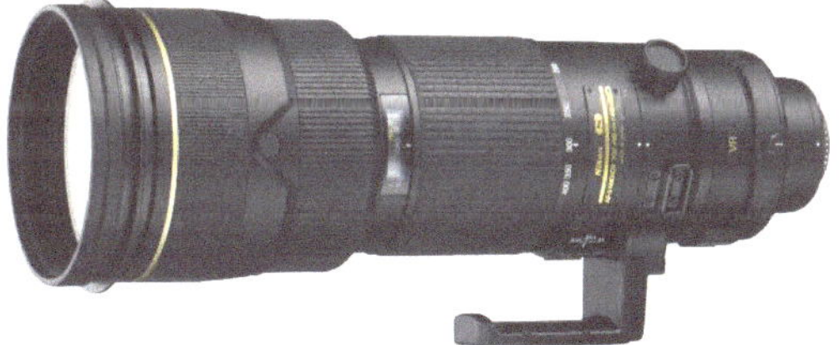

- **Wide angle lens:** When a lens has a focal length shorter than the diagonal of the negative, it is called a wide angle lens. These lenses have a larger field of view and short focal length and thus cover more of the view and the image becomes smaller and more subject – matter is included. Wide angle lenses have a much greater depth of field and are made from 17 mm to 35 mm focal length. They are very useful for creating unusual effects, while taking pictures in a narrow place and for press photography.

- **Zoom lens:** This lens is of variable focal lengths; it makes it possible to have quick change in the distance, without moving the camera. Zoom lens serves the purpose of several lenses in one, but its quality is not exactly the same as of the fixed focal length lens. Zoom lenses are mostly available from 80 mm to 200 mm, 60 to 300 mm focal length and are known ***telezooms***. Nowadays some zoom lenses are from 28 mm to135 mm focal length which serves the purpose of a wide, normal and long focus lens in one.

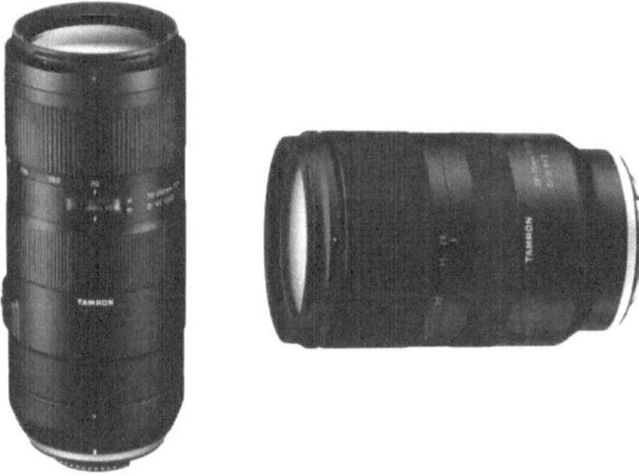

- **Macro lens:** Though this lens has the same focal length as a normal lens i.e. 50 mm, it has one additional and charming feature; it works from infinity to a close-up of 3 to 4 inches. The macro lens is also good as a normal lens and is extremely useful for close-up, nature and creative pictorial effects in general. Dental Photography: 100-105mm Macro lens.

Depending on the preference of the photographer and the situation, a wide variety of choices can be exercised in order to get the required effect from the lens.

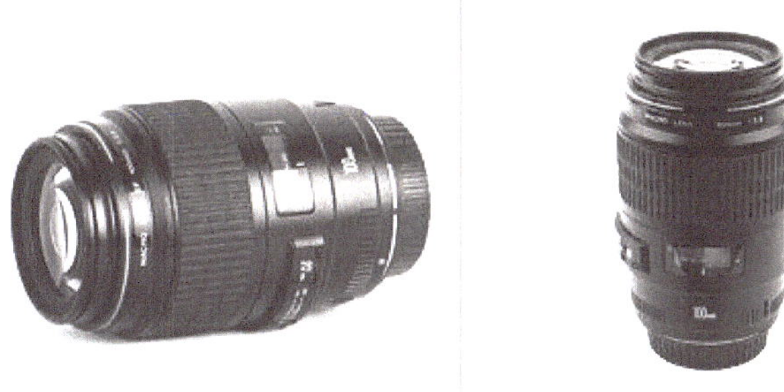

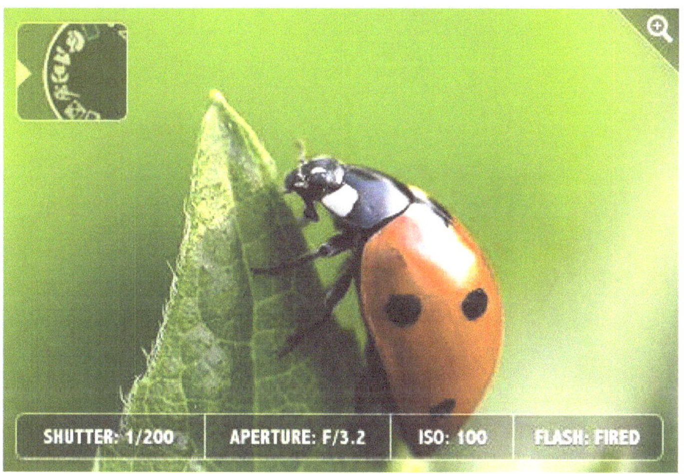

3.The shutter:*The purpose of the shutter is to protect the film from light until the chosen moment.* ***The shutter speed is the length of the exposure time.*** It is a mechanical device, which passes the light through the lens of the camera so that an image is formed on the film. In different cameras, shutters are of various kinds. Mostly they are of the following types:

a) ***Rotating metal disc with a hole*** : In box and compact type cameras

b) ***Compour shutter***, which consists of a number of overlapping steel blades. Used in twin lens reflex, range–finder and large format cameras

c) ***Focal plane shutter*** which consists of a cloth or metal blind with a moving slit. Used in most of the single reflex cameras.

These are of two types – *Mechanical and electronic*.

Mechanical - Conventional type of focal plane shutter is a mechanical shutter. Here desired shutter speed has to be set by hand before using the cameras, and there is no need of any battery to operate a camera fitted with this type of shutter. Battery is used only to operate exposure meter which is independent of the shutter.

Electronic - shutter is powered by an electromagnet and in which various shutter speeds are controlled electronically. These types of shutters operate with the help of battery which also activates exposure meter. Cameras fitted with electronic shutter cannot be operated without the battery.

4. The view-finder: The main purpose of a view – finder in the camera is to look at the subject through it, and compose the picture area before shooting. The view-finders are of the following types:

a) ***Waist level reflecting finder*** – fitted in some box cameras

b) ***Direct eye level finder***, with or without range-finder fitted in compour shutter type miniature cameras :

c) ***Ground glass and mirror view-finder*** – fitted in twin lens and in some single lens reflex cameras and

d) ***Prism, ground glass and mirror view-finder*** – fitted in most of the single lens reflex cameras.

Beside the above four main parts of the camera, there are the following *three main features of controlling the exposure and producing a sharp image.*

1) ***Aperture or stop i.e. 'f'***: *The aperture is an opening through which the light passes from the subject to the film. The aperture size is a measure of the size of that opening. It controls the amount of light that is allowed to* *pass through the lens, and eventually strike the film. The aperture does this either by opening or closing, and allowing more or less light to pass through.*

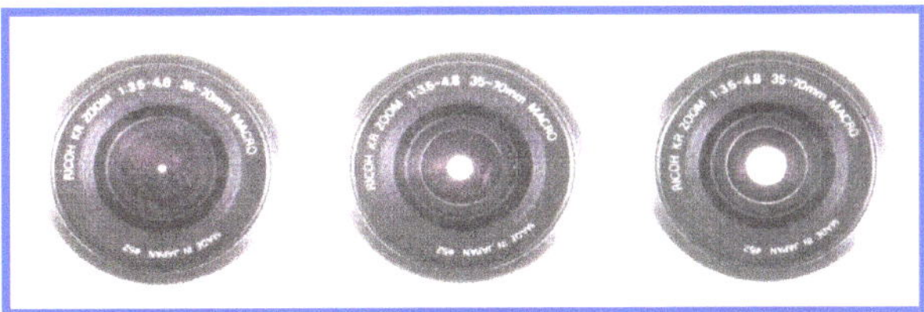

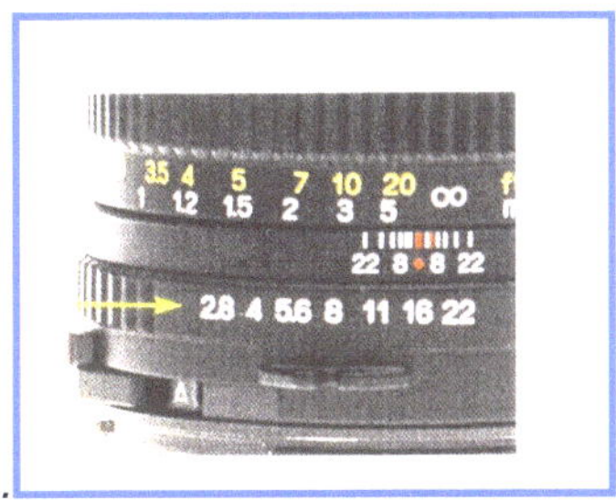

Some lenses have a rotating ring on the lens barrel called the aperture selection ring. Other cameras have an electronic dial to control this setting.

- The aperture of any lens is the ratio between the focal length and the diameter of the lens opening. The fact, the aperture system serves as a universal measurement of the light- admitting capacity of any lens and so it has a universal series which runs in this way: *f – 1.4, 2, 2.8, 3.5, 4; 5.6, 8, 11, 16. 22.* Any of these apertures can be used by setting the pointer on the appropriate number. At each setting the lens admits, twice as much light as at the next higher aperture of half as much as at the next lower aperture. It should be remembered that the highest number viz. 22 in the said series corresponds to the minimum aperture, and when the aperture is set at 22 the light passing through the lens will be the minimum. Similarly, the smallest number viz. 1.4 corresponds to the maximum aperture and at this number the light passing through the lens will be the maximum. The aperture is one of the most important factors for correct exposure.

For e.g.

- In a 50mm lens the lens is set to f/2 aperture.
- Therefore, the diameter of the aperture must be 50/2 i.e. 25mm.
- Similarly, in a 100mm lens an aperture setting of f/2 means a diameter of 100/2 i.e., 50mm

f/22 - small aperture
Deep Depth of Field
f/2.8 - large aperture
Shallow Depth of Field

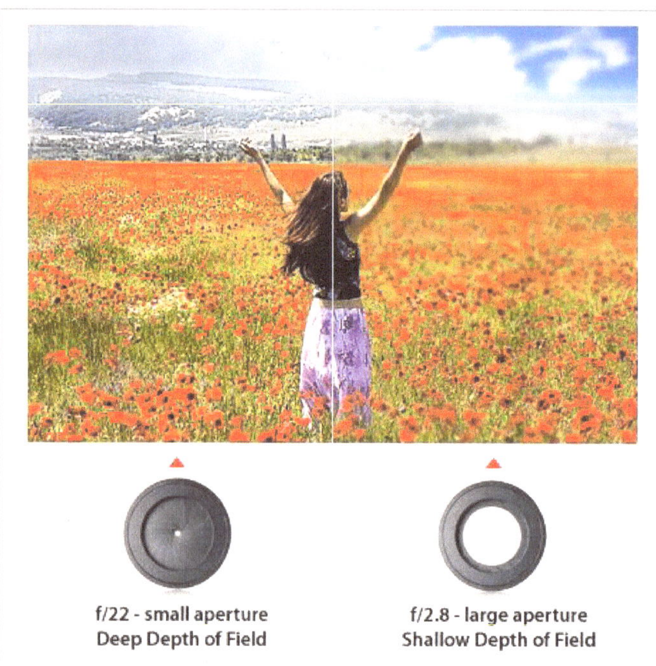

2. ***<u>Shutter speed</u>***: This is another equally important device in the camera for correct exposure of the film. The function of the shutter in a camera is two-fold.
    - First and most important function is to regulate the time during which light reaches the film; this duration of time is known as the *shutter speed.*
    - The second function of the shutter is to synchronize the flash contact.

Shutters have speeds ranging from ½ sec. to 1/8000 sec. A fast shutter speed, 1/2000 sec., 1/4000 sec., etc means that the shutter is open only for a brief moment. A slower shutter speed, 1/30 sec., ½ sec. means the opposite; the exposure is made for longer.Do not let the numbers on your camera confuse you. A shutter speed shown as '2000' means 1/2000 – meaning very fast. The fraction indicator of 1/ is left out to 'simplify' things.Each speed will allow half as much of light strike the film as the preceding one. For eg.1/30 will allow twice as much light as ***1/60 would.Usually, in Dental Photography, we have standard situations which are static. Therefore, the shutter speeds are also standard viz. 1/60***

"T" and "B" settings: T represents time exposure and is used for very long exposures. When the shutter is set close it. 'B' represents brief exposure and is used for short exposures. When the shutter is set at 'B' and pressed, the shutter opens and remains open till you release it. Nowadays in cameras, only B is designed, but in older models one comes across the T setting.

3) ***Focusing:*** Beside the aperture and shutter speed the third important control device in the camera is to set the correct distance between the lens and the object in order to get a perfect and sharp image on the film. The adjustment is called ***focusing***. Focusing is done in different types of cameras in the following three ways:

a) In many less expensive camera as it is done by just setting the distance on the lens focusing scale by guessing
b) In reflex cameras the image is seen on the ground glass screen and the lens is moved forward or backward till the image is sharp ;
c) In couple range-finder type cameras, when two split images fuse into one, the image becomes sharp.

TYPES OF CAMERA

These days several types of camera are available. In general, they can be grouped in the following categories:

1) ***Simple box camera:*** These are roll film cameras where in 120 mm, 35 mm, 110 mm size films are used.

These types of cameras are fitted with a simple small lens. Usually with a fixed aperture of f.16 or f.11. Shutter speed is also fixed e.g. 1/125 of a second. There is no focusing device in these types of cameras; any subject between four feet to infinity comes out reasonable sharp. ***These cameras are useful for taking photographs of stationary subjects in bright sunlight***.

2) ***Simple miniature camera:*** These are generally of a fairly high standard, with a number of apertures and shutter speeds. Some have a built in exposure meter or they have an electric eye to control the exposure. This eliminates the problem of setting the aperture and shutter speed for every exposure. Most of these are couple range-finder type and fitted with a compour shutter. The film size required is usually made, but still some old models are available and they usually taken 120 mm and 35 mm size films. These are also fitted with a high quality lens and some have a built-in-range-finder also. These types of cameras produce pictures of a fairly good standard. All the cameras in this category are fitted with a 50 mm normal lens for 35 mm cameras and 75 mm normal lens for 120 size cameras.

3) Compact aim and shoot 35 mm and 110 cameras:These are latest type of cameras good for snap shooting and record photography. Some are of box type and others with some additional features. These are non-interchangeable lens type cameras, fitted with 38 mm to 45 mm focal length lens or some with a zoom lens, with aperture as large as f 2.8.

In these types of cameras focusing system is of three types.

a) Cameras with fixed aperture and shutter speed works on depth of field phenomena in which usual range is from 3 or 4 feet to infinity.
b) Distance between camera and subject is guessed or estimated and fixed before exposing on a distance scale, marked on the lens.
c) Zone focusing system is available in slightly expensive cameras. Usually three to four different zones of focusing ranges are provided e.g. 3-10 feet, 10-20 ft, 20 infinity or marked as near, middle and far.

Other features of these cameras are automatic exposure control, film speed setting, winding and rewinding etc. These cameras are fitted with a compour shutter. Some models of compact cameras have a built-in flash and data back also to print day, date, year and time etc on the print. In these types of cameras minimum adjustments are needed before shooting hence they are called aim and shoot type of cameras. All the functions of these types of cameras work on two AA pen cells. Built in flash being small is good upto 10 feet distance and not beyond.

4) Modern reflex camera:The most popular cameras nowadays are the reflex cameras. These are compact, versatile and handy to use. The main feature of a reflex camera is its horizontal ground glass focusing screen on the top of the camera. The light, after passing through the lens, strikes a plane mirror placed at an angle of 45^0 to the axis between the film and the lens, thus forming an image on the ground glass horizontal screen. Focusing is done by moving the lens. The optical distancc of the lens from the film and the screen being exactly equal, a sharp image on the focusing screen is ensured, which in its turn ensures a sharp image on the film. There are two types of reflex camera ***single lens reflex*** **and** ***twin lens reflex.***

a) *Single reflex cameraLens:*

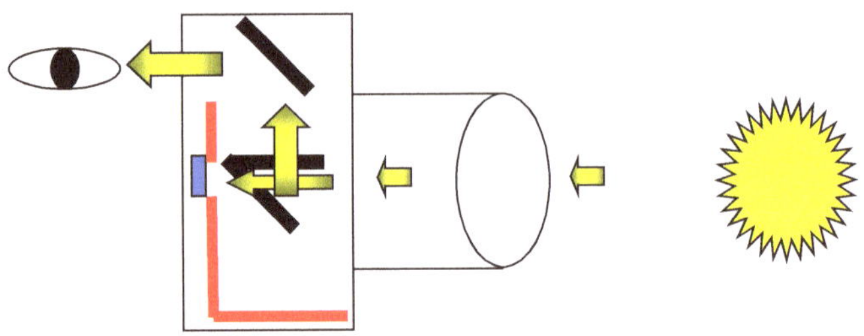

These all-purpose cameras are popularly known as *S.L.R. cameras*. Most of them produce 24mmx36 mm size negatives and some 6cm x 6cm. But they all have one common feature: *What is seen is exactly the picture in making*. This permits a perfect composition to be made, and the best possible focusing while making the picture. In S.L.R. cameras, the lens for viewing and taking the picture is the same. A front surface polished plane mirror throws the image upon a ground glass screen and prism view-finder of the same size as the negative. When the shutter is pressed, the mirror lifts up and light reaches the film. Most of the expensive S.L.R. cameras have instantaneous mirror return device, but in some less expensive cameras until the film is wound to the nextnumber the mirror does not return to its original position. The outstanding feature of a S.L.R camera is its interchangeability of lenses. Most of these take 35 mm size film, but some are of big format also and take 120 mm and 220 mm size films. The focal length of the normal lens is 50 mm or 55 mm for a 35 mm size format and 75 mm or 80 mm for 120 mm size format. Minimum shutter speed in these cameras is 1/1000 sec. and in some even upto 1/8000 sec. *35 mm S.L.R. cameras* are now available in three types. *Manual, Auto* and *Auto focus type*.

COMPONENTS OF A 35mm SLR CAMERA

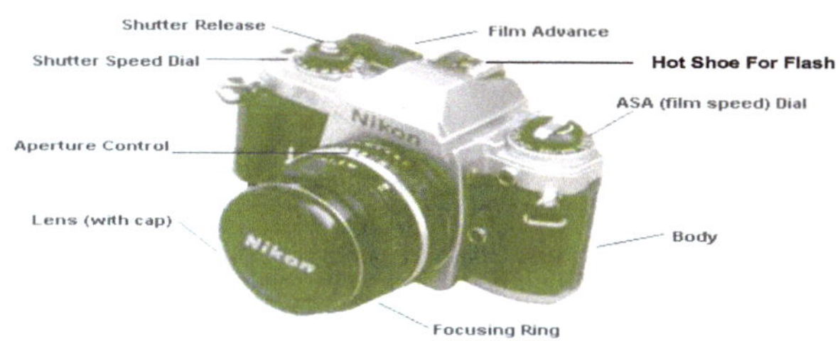

b) Twin lens reflex camera:

The second type of camera in the reflex series in the market is the twin lens reflex, an equally useful camera. This camera is good for almost all kinds of photography. In these cameras two lenses of equal focal length are mounted rigidly together with their axis parallel and horizontal. The upper lens is used for viewing and composing the picture, while the lower lens is for making the actual picture which forms the image on the film. The image appears on the ground glass horizontal screen of the view-finder (as in the single lens reflex) through the upper lens, the aperture of which always remains fully open. Twin lens reflex cameras are fitted with a compour: *shutter and the minimum shutter speed* in these cameras is either 1/300 sec. or 1/500 sec. The rim of the lens is marked with various shutter speeds from 1, 2, to 300 and 500. There is another lever which runs across a series of apertures from 2.8, 3.5, 4 to 16 and 22. All twin lens reflex cameras take either 120 mm or 220 mm size films. Some of these have an adapter-back system; hence a 35 mm size film can also be used. Lenses are not interchangeable in most of the twin lens reflex cameras, but some of these have a built-in exposure meter.

Some well-known and good twin lens reflex cameras which one can buy in India are: Rolleiflex, Rolleicord, Mamiya, Minolta, Yashica and Seagull – all in

120 mm size format. The twin lens reflex camera is very handy, all-purpose camera and worth investing money, for indoor and outdoor photography.

PHOTOGRAPHY IN DENTISTRY

PROCEDURE IN TAKING EXTRA ORAL VIEWS:

- **Selection of background**
- **Lighting for Extra-oral pictures**
- **Acc. to Proffit (extra oral views)**
  - Frontal view with lips relaxed
  - Frontal view with lips together
  - Profile view with lips relaxed
  - Profile view with lips together
  - Smile (Angular or frontal)
- **IDEAL HEAD POSITIONS (Frontal view)**
  - Outer canthus to superior attachment of the ear (C-SA line);
  - Interpupillary line;
  - Encompassing area (crown to collarbone).

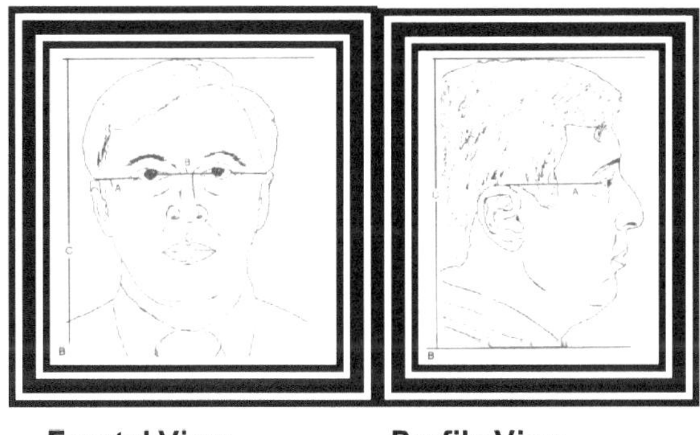

Frontal View **Profile View**

Profile view: Outer canthus to superior attachment of ear (A) and encompassing area of crown to collarbone (C).Chin and neck should show, preferably up to the clavicles. Use Frankfort horizontal line to be sure that head is levelled. The distance from outer canthus to hairline should be equal on both sides.

Oblique view: Make sure that about half of opposite upper lid eyelashes are visible andthe pupil of opposite side is not.

Smile: As broad and grin as possible, with the teeth showing.

Hairstyle: Hairstyle can distract from facial analysis. Hair should be pulled back, in a ponytail, if necessary. This allows for auricular analysis and for relationship between tragus and infraorbital rim to be evaluated. Same applies to hair down over forehead.

- Camera position for lateral view

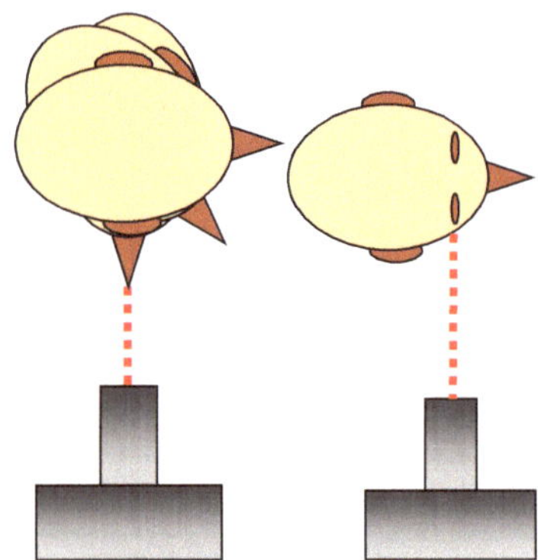

- Shadows in E/O pictures:

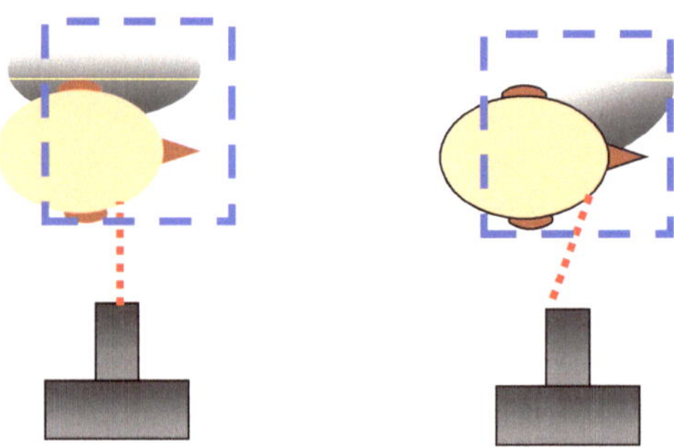

- To prevent shadows

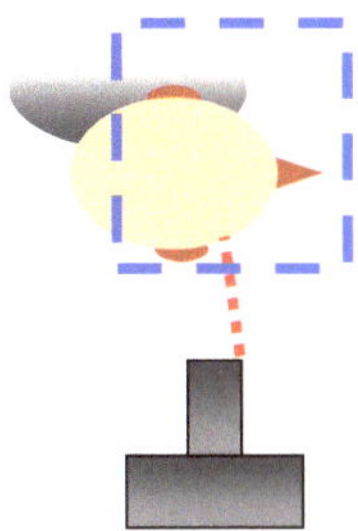

Intraoral views:

The basis of an excellent clinical photograph is clean and accurate rendering of the subject area free of visually distracting influences such as saliva or materiaalba or of the poor use of mirrors, retractors, or backgrounds. The proper position of the flash is vital to good contrast and shadow direction. Light produces the image, and its use and direction give the subject good detail and contrast. The position of the patient is important to the camera view and to the operator's ease in making the view. All intraoral views cannot be accomplished with the patient and chair in the same position. Adjust the chair height and position to satisfy the requirements of each view. For most straight anterior views, the patient should be in a semi upright position with a slight tilt backwards. In a contour chair, the patient must turn the head to the side so that the operator does not have to lean sideways over the chair and patient. The chair and patient need to be at correct height so that the operator is comfortable in using the camera.

The operator's dental light should not be directly on the teeth. With some dental operator's light, a color balance shift can be seen on the teeth and tissue. Also, in some instances, an overexposure can result. Keep the light on the side of the cheek and out of the mouth. The light is only needed to give enough light to focus by. When the dental light is bright or strong on the side of the arch that should have the greatest contrast, it will kill the contrast produced by the flash. Focus should be on the particular lesion or tooth for close-up views. For full mouth views, focus should be just ahead of half the anterio-posterior distance. In most views, this would be cuspid midline to first bicuspid midline. At this point of focus, depth of field will produce anterior-posterior sharpness. With intraoral image area or ratio selected, move the entire camera unit back and forth to the point on critical focus in the viewfinder. As the camera finder has a critical focus spot in the center, move this spot to the side to check the focus. In general use, one can also tell at the side of the finder if the bicuspids are in focus. For clinical views, do not focus with the bellows focus knob since it only changes the image ratio for from mid bellow on out to 1 to 1. Every time the bellows focus knob or the lens focus ring is moved, the image size changes, which is undesirable. Move the entire camera for focus. For intraoral views, background consideration, such as other teeth, is only important to ensure that the teeth are not in conflict with shadow, retractors, or instruments in the mouth.

The slide image should include only main points of interest. The camera should be close enough. Exchange retractors, mirror edges, fingers, and above all the patient's lips when not wanted as a part of the scene. Make sure the camera lens is set for the correct f-opening (f/22) for an area of six anterior teeth. Intraoral views for black people should use one half stop more open (f/19). The f-opening will depend on the film speed, power of the flash, and its position on the bracket. It will also be a factor when only white is to be photographed. Pure white subjects require less light, so these views should be f/27. Position the flash byrotating the bracket for the correct contrast and shadow position. Make sure the flash unit is on, and that its light shows it is ready to be fired. After exposures are made, turn the flash off to conserve the battery charge. There is no difference in exposures from battery to AC power use or Nicad battery use. Two plastic lip retractors should be used for general views. The lip retractor on the same side as the flash must be extended more than the retractor on the other side. This adjustment will keep the retractor from causing any shadow on the posterior teeth.

With all adjustments considered, to make the final exposure, move the camera forward (the automatic lens is wide open) to see the area selected. It will only be sharp in a narrow band (one tooth) as the lens is wide open. Adjust the camera altitude to the patient's position to minimize movement of the camera. Keep the arms close to the body, or rest the elbow on any handy support. With all the preceding steps performed and the full mouth area free of saliva, move the camera back away from the centrals until they are just out of focus, then move forward and focus on the cuspid or first bicuspid. Instantly squeeze the shutter's cable release in the pistol grip with a smooth action. When the lens automatically stops down to f/19 for a full mouth view, the anterior and posterior will be sharp. When and where very close-up views with critical focus are a must, more than one view should be made. The flash for all intraoral views should be at one side or the other of the lens, such as 9 or 10 o'clock or 2 or 3 o'clock and almost never at 12 o'clock, except for a direct view under the tongue.

Intraoral lighting and contrast:

With a side-mounted 180^0 rotation to the flash, the lighting and contrast can be changed for each scene. The flash should be on the correct side of the lens to produce some shadow, which gives the subject form and detailed texture. Ninety percent of all intraoral views should be made with the flash at 9 or 3 o'clock. Generally, never use the flash at 12 o'clock because it will produce shadows from the upper lip or maxillary teeth that may block out detail in wanted areas of the gingiva or oral cavity. Though in some views the flash at 12 o'clock is used that is the lower arch or under the tongue with the tongue held up. Always use the flash at 12 o'clock for objects out of the mouth.

To determine the best position of the flash for the teeth and for other details, use the following information as a guide. When the flash is mounted in the bracket close to the lens, the least amount of contrast and texture will be on the side of the arch that the flash is directed into. The opposite side of the arch from the midline will have the greatest amount of texture and shadow. If the flash is on the right side of the lens (facing the patient), the patient's left side of the arch will have the flash directed straight into the proximal spaces. The right side of the patient's arch will have the light going across the teeth, causing more shadow with the mesial lighter than the distal on each and detail. A ring-flash gives no contrast or texture in any area, which makes it a poor light source. For greater contrast to the six anterior teeth, to show enamel texture or detail, remove the flash from the bracket and hold it at a 45^0 angle so that it will cross-light the anterior teeth. When the flash is removed from the bracket, it should be held as it was on the bracket, maintaining the same distance from flash to teeth. If the distance is different, the exposure will be lighter or darker; depending upon the new distance the flash is now from the teeth. When a great amount of texture is wanted for tissue lesions or enamel wear patterns, the flash should generally be used at the 45^0 angle or greater to the subject. When this is done, make two exposures giving one of the slides a little more exposure, such as f/16 or f /19 instead of f/22. Always make enough exposures for an important area.

Whichever side of the arch the flash is directed onto will always have the least shadow or contrast, but it still will be adequate. The dentist-photographer decides where the greatest amount of contrast and detail should be. If the flash is not rotated, the slides will always have less shadow and detail of structure on the same side. Half of the time, this may cause some of the slides to have lighting that could have been better, had the proper lighting decision been made.

Retractor shapes:

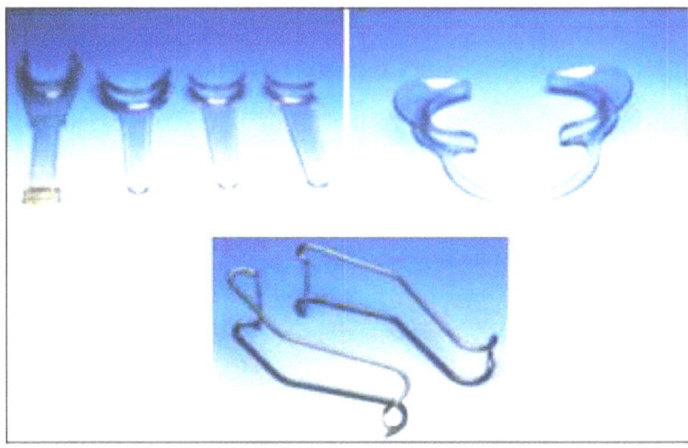

Because the size of mouths varies, more than one pair of retractors should be available. Modifying a pair of curved blue plastic retractors by cutting about 3/8 of an inch off each lip side. The retractors should then be recontoured at the ends and polished. These are ideal for use with children or a person with a small mouth. It is also recommended that a second pair be modified by cutting 3/8 inches off only one end of each retractor. With one end longer, this pair can be used to hold a large full upper or lower lip out of the way for anterior gingival views. All curved lip retractors should be single ended with stout handles. Retractors can be modified or cut down for special applications. Cleft lips almost always require modified retractors for good intraoral photography. Because the cleft lip is tight with little elasticity, a very small retractor may be a necessity. Curved metal wire retractors have some applications and should be used when needed. The main application for this retractor is buccal mirror views. For general use, curved metal wire retractors similar to the blue plastic types should not be used, since they cause glaring from their bright chrome surface. A spring loaded, self-holding, lip retractor is also very poor for photography use, as is the plastic self-holding retractor.

Application of retractors:

Unless the use of a lip retractor is going to cover the area to be photographed, two retractors should always be used. In general, a better view of the oral cavity may be obtained with two, and control of the oral cavity lighting is facilitated. If the patient's mouth is very small and the lips very tight, one retractor can be used for right or left buccal views, then a small retractor on the other side can be used just to keep the lips apart so that the flash can illuminate the area well. Sometimes this second retractor can be tongue blade, the back of a mouth mirror, or two gloved fingers. With a buccal mirror, two retractors must be used, one plastic and one wire. For general views, the selecting of two lip retractors is important in relation to the areas to be viewed. For the average patient and a straight anterior view with the teeth in centric or rest position, a standard pair of blue plastic retraction should be used. With the standard curvature of large retractors, the center fullness of the lips can be better retracted so the lip does not sag and cover the gingival margin. Of prime importance in the use of retractors is how pressure is applied to the retractors and the lips. Too often, retractors are placed on the lip, and the patient or assistant is then asked to hold them and proceeds to retract the lips by pulling the handle back towards the ears. When the handles are not held straight out or slightly forward, the buccal mucosa is pressed back onto the buccal surfaces of the teeth. For posterior views, this restricts good viewing. It can also be uncomfortable for the patient, since the ends of the retractors are pressed against the gingiva. With curved plastic lip retractors, the long, thin buccal mirror does not fit the curve of the retractor. For these views, a metal wire retractor is used on the mirror side, and a curved plastic lip retractor is held in the mouth on the opposite side.

To photograph a full maxillary arch, either with a mirror or directly, one should use as large a curved set of blue-plastic retractors as possible. Always retract evenly and hold the handles of the retractors forward to open the buccalvestibules as much as possible. Never include the retractors or lips in the camera view if they can be eliminated. For maxillary arch views with the mirror, the patient's head should be tilted upward slightly so that the camera may view the arch at about a 45^0 angle in the mirror. For direct views of this arch, the neck should be bent back, placing the head and the maxillary arch in as much of a flat plane to the camera as possible. Although this position is very uncomfortable for the patient but it does allow for good photography from a low camera position. For a direct view of the mandibular arch, the head should be upright with the mandible open as wide as possible. With the retractors holding the lower lip down and out of the way, a direct view is possible. Focus should be midway in the arch. A much better view of either arch is made with a large mouth mirror.

For orthodontic profile views of the anterior teeth in centric, the retractors must be pulled back toward the ears as much as possible. The side being photographed should have the greatest retraction; the retractor on the opposite side only keeps the lips up off the central gingival margin. By pulling the retractor back flat to the face for this view, interference by the hand holding the retractor, as well as by the retractor itself, can be minimized. Where plastic or wire retractors cannot be used for views such as a lip lesion, fingers can be used to stretch the lip or extend the frenum. For aesthetic appearance, It is recommended that finger cots be neatly rolled over the fingers that are to be in the scene, or gloves should be used.

The shape, size, and position of the retractor to be used will always vary with the area to be photographed. For most views, the blueplastic curved retractor of a standard size is best. The use of the wire retractor can spoil an anterior view by not holding all of the lip up out of the area to be viewed.

For some very hard-to-retract areas or where hospital surgery is required and cold sterilized plastic retractors cannot be used, it is possible to use one or two tongue blades, the back of a mouth mirror, or a Minnesota metal retractor. Without retractors of some type, not enough light shines into the oral cavity for good view. When mirrors are used, two retractors are always must – one Columbia wire lip retractor and one small or medium plastic lip retractor.

Mirrors:

With first-surface mirrors of varying shapes, many excellent photographs can be made of areas of the mouth that are otherwise very difficult to see. It is recommended to use the glass mirrors that have been rhodium-plated on one or both sides. Metal mirrors are not satisfactory; they have neither the brilliance nor smooth surface of a glass mirror. In general, round dental mirrors of small and medium size are not satisfactory. The very large, round, first-surface mirrors can be used, but these mirrors have the disadvantage of a polished metal edge and, since they are round, are hard to place in the chosen areas.

Glass mirrors of the correct shape and size may be purchased from the Washington Scientific Camera Company. This company has three standard mirrors, sold as the University of Washington set. Other shapes are available for special purposes. Of the different shapes available, some seem to work better for one person than another.

Every dentist doing serious photography should have two mirrors, and a third if he or she is involved in pediatric dentistry. For the periodontist, there is no. 2 or no. 2B buccal mirror. Large first-surface mirror for occlusal views is used. The same mirror can be used for maxillary and mandibular arches. Because this mirror is larger on one end than on the other, it may be used for varying arch sizes. For the very large oversized arch, the special no. 3 oversized occlusal mirror should be used. It is good for an edentulous arch. For posterior, lingual, and buccal views, a special mirror of the long narrow shape, a no. 1B is suggested. Other mirrors such as the nos. 1, 1C, 2 2B, and 2C can all be used. These mirrors should be made of double strength glass. Some pressure can be applied to it and the lip along with the metal retractors to hold the mirror slightly away from the posterior teeth. The no. 1 B mirror, being larger on one end, can also be used for lingual views in which a small oval mirror is needed or the buccal end can also be used for dental lingual views.

Buccal mirror views:

Because several buccal mirror shapes are being used, it is difficult to say what shape is best, except that the mirror should be about 1 or 1 1/8 in. wide and long enough to provide a handle, as well as extend into the mouth. The use of retractors with this mirror has been described earlier. The wire retractor must be used for all buccal views because the mirror fits to the shape of this retractor.

The buccal mirror should always be placed distally to the area to be viewed and should be held as close to a 45^0 angle to the buccal surfaces of the teeth as possible. Most of the time this angle will be less than 45^0. Sometimes, it will be much less. For all mirror views and especially buccal views, the only image that should be seen on the film is the mirror image of the teeth from half of the cuspid to the last tooth in the arch. With only this image showing the slide can be reversed and, if placed upside down, the image will resemble a direct view. Because the buccal mirror is narrow, the teeth should be well centered. If the anterior portion of the mirror is too high or too low, the image will be on a diagonal across the mirror. Also, if the mirror is rotated so it is not parallel to the teeth, the view will show more cusps or show more of the gingiva.

Posterior lingual views:

Posterior lingual and buccal mirror views are the hardest to make and require attention to all of the preceding details if good results are to be attained. Buccal mirrors are made of double strength glass therefore, they may also be used with some pressure against the tongue for good posterior lingual views. A little time spent in placing a mirror in the mouth produces excellent views of any area in the mouth. For the posterior lingual view, the mirror must be at about a 45^0angle and as far as possible from the area to be viewed. The mirror should not touch the lingual side of the last molar, but it should be close. The mirror should then angle across the arch so that it crosses over the first or second bicuspid as it comes out of the mouth.

PLACEMENT OF MIRRORS:

Maxillary Arch:

For ease in making intraoral views of the maxillaryarch, the patient's head should be slightly titled back. If the patient's head is tilted too far back, the dentist will find it harder to get the camera in a good position. While two plastic retractors are being placed on the lip and are being held by the patient, the assistant can warm the mirror to prevent fogging. All mirrors can also be kept covered on a heating pad and be always warm and ready for use. The assistant should hold the anterior edges of the mirror between the thumb and first or second finger. The finger and thumb should be as far anterior on the mirror as possible, which will keep them from appearing in the photograph. One rubber glove can be used, since the fingers have a better grasp on the mirror edge. The posterior of the mirror should rest on the distal cusps of the last tooth, with the mirror centered in the arch and held at about a 45^0 angle. In this position, a good occlusal view of all teeth in the arch can be taken. For lingual views of the six anterior teeth, this mirror or a smaller one should be held but should be placed on tooth distal to the last tooth wanted in the view. If the mirror is held at too steep an angle, a view of the nostrils will also be included. Keep in mind what is in the viewfinder is what will be on the film.

Mandibular arch:

In general, the same procedure is followed for the mandibular arch, except that the head must be tilted back far enough to allow this arch to be almost parallel with the floor when the mouth is wide open. If the patient's mouth is not opened wide, it is hard to get a good view. To keep fingers from appearing in the view, the dentist or the assistant should hold the mirror by its anterior edges. The mirror size must be large enough to accommodate the full arch. Move in close enough with the camera to cut out the retractor and mirror edge where possible. Except for children who need the small occlusal mirrors, almost every situation can then be covered by these three mirrors.

Tongue depressors:

Sometimes, the dentist must depress the side of the tongue or hold it to one side of the floor of the mouth. A regular tongue blade may be used satisfactorily to hold the tongue to one side, and the buccal mirror may also be used if a mirror or lingual view is wanted.

It is almost impossible to use one or two tongue blades to depress properly the posterior of the tongue for views of the uvula or tonsillar area. For this type of view, a small acrylic paddle 2 inches long and 1¼ inches wide should be fabricated. A toothbrush handle or a dental stimulator handle that has had the brush or stimulator cut off can be heated and bent to slightly more than a 90^0 angle.

The patient can hold this tongue depressor as far back on the tongue as he or she can tolerate, and in general it works well for most patients. For views of the top or side surfaces of the tongue, a 2 x 2-inch square of gauze may be placed around the tip of the tongue, thus allowing the assistant to secure a better hold from which to manipulate the tongue from side to side or extend it further for a better view.

Procedure for intraoral views:

- In intraoral anterior shot, assistant pulls larger ends of large retractors laterally and as far forward as possible.Raise the chair. Get in line with the occlusal plane. Distance should be adequate. Centre the lens with that of upper midline.

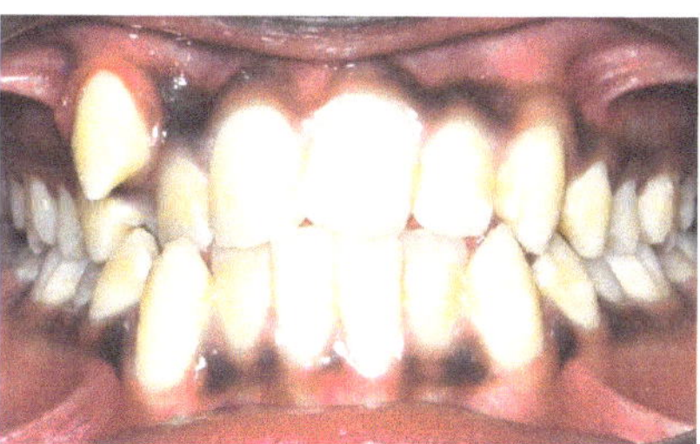

Intraoral anterior view

- Occlusal plane is horizontal. Clinically correct midline is centered. Teeth fill frame with no retractors showing.Illumination is uniform.When patient retracts the tongue, background has better contrast.

- For intraoral buccal shot, photographer holds one retractor while patient turns head as far as possible.Do not refocus. Retract more to the side than behind. Get as "side-on" as possible. Level the camera to the occlusal plane including central incisors to distal surfaces of first molars.Occlusalplane should beeven&well illuminated.Nice lateral view of the molars withminimal or no retractors showing.

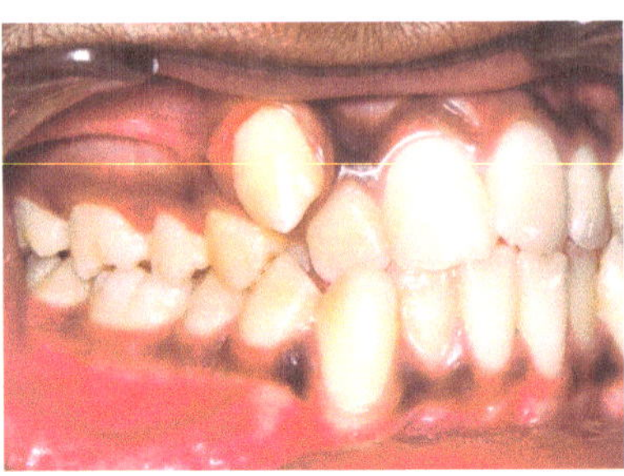

- **Upper occlusal mirror shot:**Patient tilts head back while photographer holds mirror.Assistant pulls lips upward, laterally, and forward.Keep the chair as low as possible and try to get 'on-top'.
- **Upper occlusal view:**Shot includes incisors and second molars.
- **Lower occlusal mirror shot:**Patient tilts head back while photographer holds mirror and assistant pulls lips downward, laterally, and forward.Get the chair back up & go in for straight-on position.Do not refocus after the upper occlusal shot.
- **Lower occlusal view:**Shot includes incisors and terminal molars, with no retractors or fingers visible

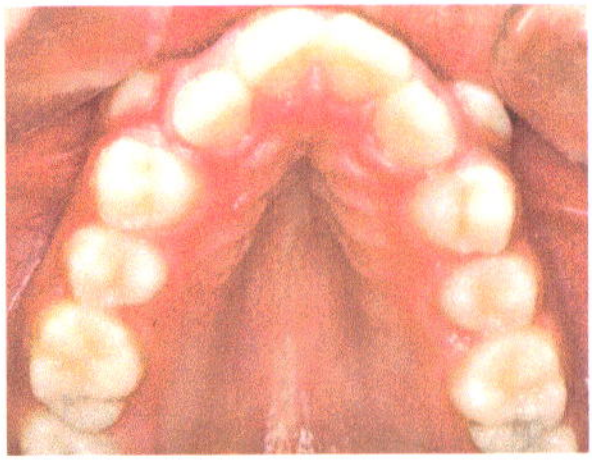

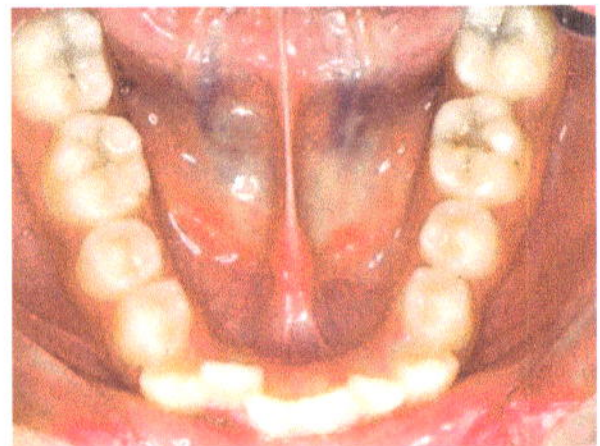

- Clean the target site of debris, excess saliva and air bubbles before taking the photograph.

- Target area should be moist but not desiccated.
- Isolate the target site (include only what is necessary in photograph)
- Use retractors as appropriate to afford an unrestricted view of the target area
- Use a high-quality mouth mirror as appropriate to view the target area.
- Control fogging by dipping mirror into hot water then drying it with a soft tissue.
- Alternatively, use a light stream of air from the air syringe to keep the mirror from fogging.
- Keep the patient's nose out of a palatal view of maxillary incisors.
- Keep fingertips, mirror edges, and retractors out of the picture.
- Camera settings remain the same
    1. f/22
    2. 1/60 sec.

FACIAL VIEWS

A 35 mm camera body and a 100 mm or 135 mm focusing lens with a Washington rotating flash bracket produces excellent facial slides or prints. The clinical camera with the 100 mm lens and bellows can also be used. A second camera for facial views may be needed if a clinical camera is used at the dental chair. The 100 mm lens will require a lens-to-subject working distance of 5 feet for the proper head size on 35mm film The camera can be hand held or fixed on a tripod or even swung out or hanging down from a wall bracket. To keep image sizes the same, a fixed distance should be marked on the floor. For hand-held shots, set the focus the same each time and move the camera body forward or back to arrive at the point of critical focus on the eyes. Do not focus the lens barrel or bellows very much, since that changes the size of the image from picture to picture. Placing a piece of tape on the focus ring prevents it from being moved.

For facial views, the camera must be held vertically. With the camera still vertical for the profile view, the flash must rotate to the side of the lens. The flash must be on the side of the lens so that the light is directed into the front of the face, casting any shadow from the profile in back of the head and out of view.

If the person is facing the camera so that the right side of his face is seen, the flash must be on the right side of the camera lens (as the camera is held). The flash above the lens for a profile view will cause a bad shadow on the background from the nose and chin. At 5 feet unless the head is smaller than normal, the back one-quarter of the head and hair, just behind the ear, will be cut off.

For a frontal view, the average head measures 8 to 8 ½ inches from ear tip to ear tip. From the tip of the nose to the back of the head, the measurement is 9 ½ to 10 inches. With these different dimensions, it is necessary to cut off about 1 ½ to 2 inches of the back of the head to keep the frontal and profile views in the same proportion.

When the dentist moves the camera back to fill the viewfinder with a profile view, the head will appear smaller. With the camera vertical and the flash used at 12 o'clock for frontal views, there will be no shadow on the background if the persons' hair at least covers his ears. The person should be 10 to 12 inches from a white colored matte surfaced background. If the hair length is shorter than the ears there will be a soft shadow below each ear. This shadow is a distraction and to eliminate any shadow, it is necessary to use a second flash on the background. When a second flash is used, the patient must be approximately 2 to 3 feet from the background.

Prefer to place the flash on a backrest or light stand so that the flash comes up onto the wall from a position midway between the patient's shoulders. The flash should be angled up onto the wall to give even illumination in back of the head. Because the distance from the flash to the wall is half that of the flash on the camera to the patient, the second or background flash could have only half the light output. In general, it is better with the same flash that is on the camera; with the same power flash on the camera that will then have a backup flash. The background flash should be connected to a slave tripper unit. With a slave tripper, when the front flash goes off to make the exposure, it activates the slave unit that causes the second flash to fire at the same time. Instead of the slave tripper, a long flash extension cored can be used but, in general, it is always in the way.

Floodlights on a background are hot, and unless they are blue, they are the wrong color of light for use with daylight film. Fluorescent tube backgrounds or viewing screens can be used. Make sure they are the correct color balance for daylight film if white background is required. It will do no good to use filters on mixed lighting, as light will always be of wrong color.

When the background light is not strong enough, a longer shutter exposure is necessary even when the flash is used on the front. This longer shutter exposure will burn out a background shadow; but, with the slower shutter speed, if the patient moves after the flash has gone off, there are now two exposures, and one is blurred, prefer the single flash in the proper position and the patient 10 or 12 inches from a white background there will be no background shadow unless the person's ears are not covered by hair. Even then, the shadow is very soft and slight. The further the patient is from the background, the more shadow there will be, and the darker the background will be.

When making frontal or profile views, most dentists give very little consideration to the height of the camera lens and its relation to the patient's face. For good photographic drawing to render the subjects true to natural as possible, the dentist should aim the centre of the lens 1 to 1 ½ inches above the pupil of the eye. Looking down or up to any great degree with the camera lens will distort the patient's facial features. As stated earlier, the 100- or 135-mm lens is best suited for all types of facial views. The background can be any material that is not glossy. Prefer a white matte or dull-finished wall. A white mounting board can also be used, or a painted window shade can be pulled down and used. Black or dark backgrounds should not be used, since dark hair will blend with the dark background and leave only the face visible. Facial views of patients in a dental chair are generally poor. The photographs will have no background or will show the floor or wall cabinets or chair headrest.

For a profile view of the patient, remember that the patient's face must be rotated 3 to 5^0 back toward the camera lens. The reason for this is lens optics. From a single lens viewpoint, objects that have a third dimension appear to be turned away from the lens on the outside edge. With a profile view, and the camera pointed at the center of the head, the face appears to be turned away from the camera. An easy guide to a 3^0 to 5^0 rotation is to have the patient turn toward the camera just so that the edge of the backside of the eyebrow can be seen. The outline of the distal central can also be used. A second way to arrive at a true photographic profile is to shift the camera to the side so the lens is pointed at the corner of the eye, rather than at the ear. One still must cut off the back quarter of the head to give the proper head sizes for both views.

BACKGROUND AND LIGHTING FOR OBJECTS:

Many clinicians need to photograph small objects such as extracted teeth, impressions, casts, biopsy specimens, bands, and so forth. The clinical cameras will photograph these objectswell, provided the dentist knows how to show the subject to its best advantage.

BACKGROUND:

Most dentists use the first piece of cloth, paper, or tabletop that is handy and do not think about what the background does visually to the subject. The texture or lack of it and color are most important when selecting a background. Next in importance is how the background is to be used, such as a flat sheet of paper or one curved to form a floor and a wall without a crease in the paper (which eliminates a line of horizon). For direct anterior views of casts, the background can curve over the front edge (two or three inches) of the counter or table.Again, the gentle curve up from the tabletop to form a back wall. Again, the gentle curve eliminates a line of horizon. With the camera lens lined up along the cusps of the teeth, all three surfaces of the background will blend together for a smooth clean background. In general, for most objects, use the background paper flat and curved up in back instead of just a flat piece of paper. A flat piece of pastel colored typing paper is good only when one is photographing almost straight down onto it. The reason for the curved paper is that a back wall for the object is formed in this way. This wall, providing it is not too far away from the object, the background floor or base therefore the background will not trail off and be dark as the flash diminishes by the distance the light must travel.

Paper for a background is inexpensive and when soiled or wrinkled, it can be discarded. The paper should be smooth and dull without any glossy finish. For close-up views of burrs or other instruments, paper without any texture at all is the best. For full mouth casts or other objects, where a colored background is required, crepe paper can be stretched to take out the wrinkles and taped down. Its texture will not prove a problem except at 1 to 1 magnifications of small objects.

Another good paper surface to use is school construction paper (use in kindergarten), or inexpensive colored typing paper is fine. For very large areas, a big sheet of brown wrapping paper makes a good background or even butcher paper can be used. The color of any background for color photography should be a light pastel. Dark colors or vivid colors become very distracting and distract from the importance of the subject. Dark and vivid, or intense colors, always become dark on film and in general do not look good.

Where a black background is wanted for white casts or other reasons, a suede or velour finish paper can be purchased from a display supply store. Black paper should be jet black, not just a black – grey.

Cloth does not make a good background because it has too much texture. Velvet can be used, but it is expensive, marks easily and shows lint. When a damp cast is placed on it, velvet will pucker or mark. A4 x 4 gauze or waffle weave bib, office towels, and countertop or wood grain patterns are poor backgrounds. All of these materials “overwhelm” the subject because of a busy background. When nothing else seems available for a background, use a piece of inexpensive white or buff typing paper or a piece of brown wrapping paper. The background should be smooth and free of wrinkles, because these are very distracting in enlarged views on a screen.

PHOTOGRAPHY OF RADIOGRAPHS

Black and white x-ray duplicating film can also be used, but most dentists have color film in their cameras. Use the standard x-ray medical view box of chest size that has two or three daylight fluorescent lamps in it. With fluorescent lamps, a 0.05 or 0.10 magenta gelatincolor correction filter must be used over the camera lens. If the filter is not used, the color slide of the x-ray film will be blue-green, which is not a bad color, and some people use it for colored slides of x-ray films. A glass FL-D filter can also be used but the cost is more than most filters. The FL-D filter can also be used, though for a view of areas that have all fluorescent lighting.

Place the radiograph to be copied on the view box. Mask the radiographs at least 1 inch on each side to exclude the light around the sides. If a radiograph is not masked, such as a large film of the head, then be sure that no white light is seen in the camera view finder. This light will cause a poor exposure. Place the camera directly over the radiograph by using a copy stand or a crank-up tripod, or stand the view box on end, and shoot directly into it. With the camera on a center column crank-up tripod, place the camera bellows on a focusing rail, then onto the tripod.

Adjust the bellows for an image ratio of 1 to 1 or to the size of the radiograph and focus on it. The focusing rail makes 1 to 1 copy much easier to do. If it is not used, move the entire tripod back and forth on the floor to focus. Use a camera with a built – in meter to make a reading of the light through the radiograph.

Because of the bellows, one must know how to use the meter through the bellows. It can be done easily. Reset the shutter speeds to a setting of one second or one half second and make sure the lens is wide open and on manual operation. For Minolta units, activate the manual preview set button. If the radiograph is dark or very dark, the view box may not have enough light to give a meter reading. A flash unit may be necessary. The room light should be off so the meter is only measuring the transillumination, on top-reflected light off the radiograph.

From the correct exposure on the meter with the lens and shutter set, the exposure with a cable release is made so that the camera is not moved. Exposure examples for K64 film and through the bellows metering will depend on the light output of the view box and the density of the radiograph. Most exposures will be made at one half second or one second, at a lens opening of f/5.6 to f/8. If the radiograph has a great amount of contrast, the metering will not be correct because of the clear area in the film. One full stop more exposure must then be added from what the meter says.

When copying a radiograph with the flash unit, it is best to use a center column crank-up tripod with a bellows-focusing rail for fine focus. The focusing rail for Minolta attaches to the bottom of the bellows I. With a tripod, the slides can be critically framed. Place the radiograph on a piece of white Plexiglas 1/8 x 11 x 14 inches – the white plastic # 2447. Put the plastic on edge in a 1/8-inch slot in a 2 x 4 inch or a 2 x 6-inch base 6 inches long. The base will support the plastic upright. Tape the radiograph on the plastic with black 1-inch-wide photographic tape. Mask off the radiograph if the photograph is going to go to the edge. If the radiograph is already mounted and forms a mask, leave it as it is. With the radiograph on the plastic and the camera on a tripod as described, set the bellows for a 1 to 1 image of one bite wing film. Move the camera lens about 8 inches in front of the radiograph. A light source such as a gooseneck lamp or office dental light or even the light from a slide projector in back of the radiograph is necessary. With the focus rail, one can move the entire camera back and forth. Camera bellows can be used to change the image size. When the image is focused, turn off or remove the focusing light and place the flash unit from the clinical camera 6 inches behind the single radiograph to be copied. The flash must be on a 6 ft PC-PC extension cord. Before the exposure is made, overhead room lights or other light sources that could put excess surface light on the face of the radiograph should be turned off.

The flash distance in back of the radiograph should be 6 inches for single films or 2 inches greater than the longest dimension of a full mouth survey or any other large size film. For a 1 to 1 copy of a normal density periapical film with a flash 6 inches behind the glass and radiograph, the exposure should be about f/11. For a first test, one should also use f/16 and f/8. The shutter must be set for a flash exposure 1/60 second. When the flash is moved back to cover a large film, the lens f-opening will remain the same. In general, the transillumination of a radiograph will require two f-openings larger than the same object image size with the light from the front by the lens on to an average dental object. When any radiograph is darker or denser, open the lens's f-stop to f/9, f/8, f/6.3 and so on. If the radiograph is very light or thin in density, close the lens's f-stop down to f/13, f/16, f/19 and so on. The flash will produce the best color balanced copy of a radiograph because it is matched to the film and in general will require no color correction filter other than what is on the flash and lens for intraoral use with K64 film. For most average density radiographs, f/11 will be the correct exposure, or very close to it. Kodak direct positive Panchromatic 5246 film gives good black and white positive slides. One problem is finding someone to process it. For truly black and white radiographs, one should use Panatomic X black and white film, develop the negative, and print it on fine grain positive. Also, 35 mm x-ray duplicating film (# SO-185) can be used in the camera when a flash is not used, but this very slow film requires exposure of up to 45 seconds or more. It can be developed in chemicals for dental x-ray film. Generally, for most dentists, the use of K64 color film for the copying a radiograph is satisfactory and is the easiest to do with the flash unit. Several other different light sources can be used for copy work, but always make sure the color of the light used is in correct color balance for the film used.

DIGITAL PHOTOGRAPHY

The buzzword today is 'digital'. Be it music, T.V., video, watch, diary or any appliance. The world is going digital.

Film less photography, pictures on a chip, call it what, this is a new phenomenon of technology. It is big and it is the way things will be from now on.

For over 160 years, photography has been based on the silver halide film, which is now being replaced.

Digital photography has come about as a result of convergence of both IT and photography. And it has so much to offer.

Now get set to explore the delightful world of digital photography and this of course requires the willingness to learn the new stuff.

Advantages:

- The major advantage going digital besides being film less and hence cost effective is that the digital pictures can be viewed and the results can be confirmed immediately, simply by hooking onto a TV or a computer.
- Images can be improved, color can be balanced, or for graphic artist the images can be manipulated with more freedom of artistic expression with no limitation to stretch the creative ability, it can also get abused in the wrong hands.
- Images can be stored, in the computer itself or on a CD. Image can be viewed in the monitor, the digital album. (Inexpensive storage)
- No wet processing is involved which also eliminates the dust and re touching procedures.
- Since photos are stored electronically, there is no ageing of photos
- This also makes retrieval easy and printouts whenever required can easily be obtained using ink jet printers.

- Some cameras have video output for TV display. Some can even capture video, which are very helpful for multimedia presentations (slight sound and motion), the comments can be recorded about the picture which are recorded as wave files.
- Transmission via the internet to across the world is feasible.
- It is versatile and allows the transfer of images between many kinds of devices and applications.

Understanding the Basics:

- Just like a conventional camera, it has a series of lenses that focus light to create an image of a scene. But instead of focusing this light onto a piece of film, it focuses it onto a semiconductor device that records light electronically.
- A computer then breaks this electronic information down into digital data.
- To do this, the image needs to be represented in the language that computers recognize – bits and bytes. Essentially, a digital image is just a long string of 1s and 0s that represent all the tiny colored dots -- or pixels -- that collectively make up the image.

THE COMPUTER:

- A computer is a necessity as a part of the photography gear and clinical armamentarium. What is the desired configuration?
- Any basic computer will do for clinical photography work, instead of wasting a major part of the budget in the fastest processor available, say a mid-range processor like a Pentium II will do. Present basic hard disk is now a 2 MB is more than what is required, display adapters, 8 MB ram, 17" monitor and say 128 MB RAM and a windows operating system.

Software:

Plenty of softwares are available for enabling the photographs to be touched up to catalogue to store and to retrieve the images.

Simple software come as freebies while buying the camera itself.

Professional practice management soft wares can be expensive but that will be bundled with other facilities like maintaining records, appointment, growth prediction, and analyses etc.

THE DIGITAL CAMERA:

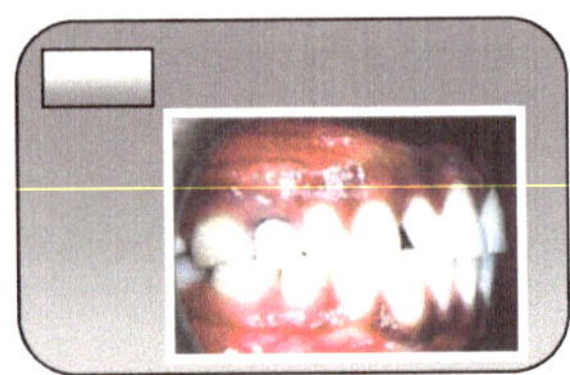

The basic first

- In conventional photography, the images of objects are recorded on film through chemical reactions with light.
- In the case of digital photography, the formation of images is identical with the systems of conventional photography- but what is different is the recording system. It is an electromagnetic reaction of light on an electronic device that captures images.
- The pictures taken are captured electronically and stored inside the camera in what is called a memory card.
- Hence this piece of equipment enables to capture the picture without a film and view it immediately in the camera itself or admire it in the monitor or TV.

How does it do that?

- The electronic device in the camera (the perpetual film) could be either a "Charged couple Device" (CCD) or a "Complementary Metal Oxide Semiconductor" (CMOS).
- These sensors are made up of tiny pixels that change light and colour into electronic computer code by means of sophisticated analog/digital processing and conversion.
- Basically, the CCDs are comprised of rows of thousands of extremely light sensitive picture elements or pixels analogous to the silver halide particles on film.
- CCD has millions of pixels arranged in a grid pattern like graph paper and can capture the whole image instantaneously, like film.

(Area array camera)

- The CCD is a semiconductor storage device where an electrical charge is moved across by signals. The presence or absence of charge denotes one or zero.
- CCDs are monochromous hence can detect only black or white, one-shot color is generally achieved with what is called a striped array. This involves filtering the individual pixels on the area array, alternating with red, green and blue.
- In fact, the CCD chip in the digital camera is a triple – decker sandwich, a bottom slab consisting of silicon, with the CCD grid spread across it. The cells in the CCD layer correspond to the pixels of light, which determines how sharply the picture is recorded on top of a filter bank, which divides the light coming from the scene into the three primary colors red green and blue, and diverts it into the corresponding CCD cells.
- There are 256 gray shades, and varying a level of each of the three colors results in the gamut of 16.7 million colors.

IMAGE STORAGE (MEMORY CARDS)

- At most all newer models have removable storage media, though the older models have built in storage.
- A removable card helps to replace cards when it is full and insert another.
- The capacity of the memory card can vary 2 MB to 64 MB and can be of different types like the smart media, compact flash cards, memory sticks pc cards or even regular floppies from which one can transfer images to the computer using adapter card reader and do the manipulation and storage of the image there.
- The card reader could be plugged into serial port, parallel ports or USB ports

Since each image will consume a considerable amount of camera's memory, a provision is made to compress the image usually in the JPEG format. This can reduce the storage space, and make the downloading faster and supports 24 bit color unlike other formats like GIFT which support 8 bits (256 colors)

It has to be noted that digital photography need not begin from digital cameras only but can also be produced from regular prints or films by digitizing them using scanners.

THE RESOLUTION:

Before really getting technical, one has to understand that the eye is incapable of discriminating details below a certain level, hence very printed picture is an image composed of dots of ink, ranging from 70 – 300 dpi.

- Digital images obey the same laws.
- If resolution is low; dots (pixels) are seen.

BIT MAP:

Image contains many individual pixels with each pixel containing a colour.

e.g.: 1 bit – black and white,

4 bit – each pixel one of 16 colour values.

THE RESOLUTION:

It is the fineness of the details of the image.

The resolution of an image is assessed in terms of the amount of pixels that make up the image. This is generally given as horizontal and vertical numbers.

This depends on the capacity of the sensors present in the camera as mentioned. That is in terms of its number of pixels (picture elements)

A digital image has no absolute size or resolution, all it has is certain number of pixels in each dimension. Now as the image size changes, the resolution changes and the same number of pixels are spread over a greater or lesser area i.e. larger print at lower quality, smaller print at higher quality.

It is obvious that more the number of pixels the better is the resolution, though that is not the only criterion for comparison.

(other components of image quality include bit depth and tonal range, colour accuracy, generational quality, consistency etc.)

1 million pixels=1 mega pixel (10,00,000 pixels per image)

640 x 480 – good enough for web publishing and presentation

The resolution is 640 x 480 = 307,200 pixels

However, this can produce small images on print say 4 x 6

For 4 x 6 prints → 640 x 480 (0.31 mega pixels)

For 5 x 7 prints → 1024 x 768 (0.79 mega pixels)

For 8 x 10 prints → 1280 x 960 (1.2 mega pixels)

11 x 14 prints → 2048 x 1536 (3.15 mega pixels)

2240 x 1680 (3.76 mega pixels)

The mega pixel camera came to existence just a couple of years ago.

[35 mm film is supposed to contain about 25 million pixels .... Still a long way for competition with the film photography]

What resolution is needed? How big is big enough?

It depends on the final hard copy. Eg: For images on screen, only 72 ppi are needed. More is just a waste. Unnecessarily a large file size makes download slower.

It looks no different on screen.

PPI and DPI : Frequently used inter-changeably by pros and amateurs alike. While wrong, it isn't a huge problem.

The correct term in scanners, digital cameras and screens are all measured in PPI, while printers are measured in DPI.

Just so to know the difference, sophisticated electronic chip (sensor) takes the place of a film for recording the image.

Note: One can increase the number of pixels in Photoshop to any size, these new pixels (empty pixels) are invented by Photoshop by one of the three methods (ressing up).
Similarly one can res-down an image say for the web – need only 72 dpi. When it is resampled, photoshop throws away unneeded pixels.

COLOUR DEPTH:

Number of colors an image has or no of tones an image has in case of gray scale.

BIT DEPTH:

Bit is a smaller unit of data. 1 or 0, on or off.

8 bite – byte (represents 256 different states).

Most of the digital world operates on 8bit images (monitor, printer, etc.)

While speaking of 8 bit images – we are calling about one that consists of 3 colors, also referred to as 3 x 8 = 24 bit image.

8 bits represents a single color.

Most cameras today have a 24 bitcolor depth (16.7 million shades) and the high – end cameras are capable of producing 36 bit depth. There are 42 and 48 – bit depths in highly professional digital back for medium and large format cameras.

TYPES OF DIGITAL CAMERAS:

1) Consumer point and shoot cameras:
   - Fully automatic
   - Have low resolution
   - 4 x 6 inches

The recent plethora of mass – marketed digital cameras, such as Apple's Quick Take, Kodak's DC series, etc. Although these cameras may be adequate for small reproduction in newsletters or web pages, they won't meet the needs of professional photographers. These consumers – level cameras use small chips with striped arrays and have a limited range of tones and colors.

2) Prosumer cameras
   - Based on the 35 mm model
   - Have well over one million pixels. They usually have good features like macro mode, LCD screen and have range finder like viewing system and not SLR model, hence generally they cannot be used for serious clinical photography. The other major problems being the facility to use additional systems like the ring flash.

3) Professional cameras

Professional class digital cameras are built on 35 mm camera bodies that use conventional interchanges lenses. Most are conversions of popular film cameras while a few are designed to be digital from the ground up.

They are called multi pixel camera as the big advantage of these cameras lies in the fact that they are SLR and hence accessories like macro lenses, ring flash etc. can be used.

Like the Nikon D1, or the Fuji Fine Pix besides being heavy they are too expensive with the body alone costing around a couple of lakhs.

Though there is an initial expense involved there is a considerable amount of savings; after a while the photography will be free.

What is good for Orthodontists?

The professional cameras with ideally a 105 mm macro lens for both intra oral and extra oral photography are used.

If the cost and great pictures are considered then one can go for a 2-mega pixel SLR model that has macro or close focus facility or else the camera that accepts close up lens.

OLYMPUS 2500 is a good compromise

It also has a small color monitor for viewing the scene one intends to capture.

There is also provision for reviewing images that the camera has in memory, which only gives a rough idea, and one can't actually access the quality of the image.

Poor images can be deleted then and there.

Most DC has 2 or 3 settings usually called normal resolution and high resolution (better referred to as poor resolution and better resolution).

One should buy a camera that has an optical viewfinder. It's cool composing with the LCD on the back of the camera.

Most come with a zoom lens (wide angle normal to tele) usually specified by

its magnification for e.g. A 3 x will enlarge or reduce by three times.

The camera usually transforms the picture into one of the industries –

standard image file formats which store the picture as a bit map: TIFF, JPEG,

EPS and PCAX, to bring up the picture on the screen and manipulate it.

DISADVANTAGES:

- Most DC's suffer momentary delay from time.

- The button is pushed until the photo is captured and even longer delay until the next photo due to memory write process.
- So not as quick and hence, no multiple rapid sessions –not for action photography.
- Chews battery like crazy especially with digital display.
- Initial cost in heavier than similar film cameras

Digital imaging, one of the hot fields in the computer world, is attracting more and more interest among orthodontists. It is now possible, with a reasonable investment, to digitally acquire, archive, and easily retrieve clinical images of our patients.

The hardware involved includes flatbed scanners; slide scanners, video cameras, digital cameras. Digital cameras can be divided into two main groups: compact digital cameras and professional reflex cameras with digital interface. The compact cameras range in price from $300 to $1,500, while reflex cameras start at a minimum of $5,000. Further, it is expected compact cameras with better performance in the same price range, as well as less expensive reflex cameras.

If the budget allowsbuying a professional reflex camera, it will certainly meet all the requirements for clinical orthodontic photography. The choice of a compact camera can be difficult, due to the wide range of quality and price. Many mistakes can be made in selecting the appropriate system for an orthodontic practice.

Optical system quality for macrophotography:

For intraoral photography, the lens system should allow adequate magnification at a distance at 12” from the subject. Shorter distances are of little use to the orthodontist. The optical quality depends on the camera’s focal length – the distance (in millimeters) between the image sensor and the optical center of the lens when the lens is focused on infinity.

Manufacturers of digital cameras usually do not indicate the actual focal length, but rather its equivalent on a 35 mm camera. For example, a focal length of 5 mm on a digital camera is equivalent to36 mm on a 35 mm camera. Many compact digital cameras have lens systems with the focal length of 36 mm (equivalent to a 35 mm camera). This value is inadequate for orthodontic intraoral photography. A 50 mm focal length will completely satisfy the requirements for dental photography. A high focal length allows a reasonable distance from the subject, minimizes distortion, increases depth of field, and permits adequate illumination of the subject.

Cameras with a zoom function have a variable focal length, which is expressed as a range. Focal length can be increased with a zoom lens or by the addition of close – up lenses. The best digital cameras have a zoom with a high magnification ratio and the ability to add close – up lenses.

When the zoom is moved toward the maximum enlargement position, or close – up lenses are added, it can become impossible to focus from short distances, and the effectiveness of the autofocus is reduced. Thus, the image in the viewfinder has a high magnification but is out of focus. The balance of these factors is what determines the macro capabilities of the system.

The macro quality of a digital camera is acceptable to capture a 70 mm horizontal line at full screen, in sharp focus, from a distance of 12". This corresponds roughly to the 1:2 magnification on a conventional 35 mm camera one of the most common magnification ratios in orthodontic photography. Many compact digital cameras, however, do not achieve this quality.

Higher macro capabilities can be useful for 1: 1.7 or 1: 1.5 magnification ratio. A very good optical system allows a 35 mm line to be captured a full screen, which corresponds to a 1:1 magnification ratio.

Autofocus speed and precision:

It is important to test the autofocus of a camera, taking into account the magnification ratio, distance from the subject, and illumination. Since the autofocus might not work properly under some orthodontic conditions, the availability of a manual focus is a plus.

A satisfactory autofocus for orthodontic purposes will work properly at a distance of 12" from the subject with a 1:2 magnification ratio.

CCD resolution and quality:

In digital photography, traditional film is replaced by a charged coupled device. A CCD sensor has thousands of light detectors, called “Pixels”, on its surface. A high number of pixels (“Optical resolution”) increases the quality and detail of the image, but also increases the size of the file in which the image will be saved.

File resolution can be increased by a software interpolation, which does not actually improve the image quality. Therefore, when evaluating a camera's optical resolution, the interpolation resolution should not be considered, but only the actual CCD optical resolution.

Some digital cameras allow an image to be captured at two or more different resolutions: the highest is the full CCD resolution, but the lower resolutions use only a portion of the CCD pixels to describe the image. This division can save file space if the CCD has a high optical resolution.

High resolution can only be used to full advantage when nothing extraneous to the required area is captured in the frame. An intraoral picture taken at a resolution of 832 x 624 meaning that about 520,000 pixels are used to describe the subject. However, the clinically useful area is displayed by only 212,000 pixels. If the image has been taken at the maximum possible magnification for the camera, then the latter number represents the “Clinically useful resolution” (CUR) for the camera.

The CUR a key factor in the choice of digital cameras, depends on both the sensor resolution and the quality of the optical lens system. A new generation of compact digital cameras with sensor resolutions of as many as 1,000,000 pixels are now in the market, but they have poor optical systems that diminish their CUR. The CUR also depends on the needs of the user. If the photograph of dental crown anatomy in detail in needed, a high CCD resolution and / or a powerful lens system will be required.

A CUR of about 400,000 pixels should be adequate for orthodontic use. It is recommended selecting a camera with a CCD resolution close to the CUR. Too great a difference will produce unnecessarily large files and thus will require more memory and a longer transfer time to the computer. If the CCD resolution is much larger than the CUR, it will be necessary to manipulate (crop) each file on the computer to avoid archiving unwanted information.

The sensor quality of a single pixel in transmitting the luminance (brightness) and chrominance (color hue) of the light signal should be tested by observing the images captured by the digital camera on a properly tuned monitor. Some CCDs show a minor shift in hue toward one of the base colors (red, green, or blue). This problem has a limited impact on image quality, since it can be easily corrected with any imagining software.

Flash capability:

In conventional dental photography, a synchronized ring flash is needed to obtain uniform illumination of the subject in macro mode. External light sources cannot be used, because the lips and chin, the camera, and the operator (whatever is close to the subject) will create shadows.

Most compact digital cameras have built – in flash units on one side of the lens. Which will produce uneven light distribution in intraoral photography and have no ports for external synchronized flash units. Even a camera with a connection for a synchronized flash may not allow the use of a ring flash, because it will cover the autofocus sensor. The ability to use a ring flash is therefore an important point in selecting a digital camera.

If the camera does not permit the use of a ring flash, the subject illumination can be improved in two ways:

1) Light deflectors a mirror system can effectively diffuse the flash light on both sides of the subject. Light deflectors for some digital camera models are currently in the market.
2) Light – activated external flash. It may be possible to mount an external flash on the opposite side of the built – in flash. The two flashes will operate simultaneously, producing good illumination of the subject without shadows.

Viewfinder:

An optical reflex viewfinder is ideal, because it provides an almost perfect correspondence between the image seen in the viewfinder and the captured image under all conditions.

An alternative is a liquid crystal displayviewfinder. The LCD can be as small as 5" in this case an optical system allows proper magnification with the eye in close contact with the viewfinder, as with most video cameras. An LCD can also be a small screen, 1.5 – 2.5" in diameter, in this case the camera must be held away from the eye when shooting. Most LCDs have a low "refresh rate", meaning that as the camera is moved to frame the best picture, the image in the viewfinder changes jerkily. Other disadvantages are that an LCD is hard to read in bright sunlight, and that a large unit consumes a great deal of battery power.

Digital cameras with Galilean viewfinders are difficult to use, because in macro photography the area framed by the viewfinder will be quite different from the one framed by the lens.

Immediate review of recorded images:

This is one of the most important advantages of digital cameras over conventional cameras. The recorded image can be checked a few seconds after taking the picture and decide whether it is satisfactory. If not, it can be deleted immediately from the camera memory and another shot can be taken.

Tuning of exposition parameters:

In macro photography, it is important to be able to manually adjust the exposition parameters: the size of the lens opening (aperture), indicated by the f-number, and the shutter speed measured in fractions of a second. It is often difficult for the automatic mechanism to function properly at close distances, particularly if the flash is used, as is often the case with intraoral photography.

Batteries and AC connection:

Some digital cameras use ordinary alkaline batteries and have a battery life of only 10-15 photographs. Others have rechargeable batteries that can last through more pictures. If the digital camera comes with two rechargeable batteries, one will never experience the “no battery” situation.

An external AC connection can be helpful even if it is not used routinely. The power cord tends to interfere with operator movement, and a socket must be available nearby.

File format and software compression:

Once an image has been acquired by the CCD, it is stored in the camera’s memory as a file. Image files can be of different formats and more importantly, can be compressed. Compression increases the number of images that can be stored in memory, but it also causes a decay of the image quality; the higher the compression, the greater the decay.

A good feature is the ability to choose whether the images are to be saved with or without compression, and at which compression level. Selecting the capture mode as "FINE" usually does this. "NORMAL", or "ECONOMY" (the terms may vary depending on the camera model).

The file storage format is not critical, but it is preferable to use digital cameras that save the acquired images as JPEG or TIFF files, which can be read virtually by any imaging software. Proprietary file formats will require special software.

Number of images stored in memory:

There are two types of image storage: built – in (internal) memory and removable memory. Digital cameras with only internal memory should be avoided. Removable memory is like a conventional roll of film that can be used over and over again. Four types of removable memory are currently available for digital cameras:

- Solid state floppy disk card (SSFDC) or "smart card".
- Miniature card
- Compact flash card
- 3.5" floppy disk

SSFDCs can store only as much as 8 MB of data, while miniature cards store as much as 24 MB. These two media need a converter that is inserted in a floppy disk or PCMCIA drive.

Compact flash cards can be found in sizes from 2MB to more than 100 MB and do not need an adapter for insertion in a PCMCIA drive. Floppy disks are inexpensive and easy to use, but have a storage capacity of only 1.4 MB.

The amount of space taken by one image depends on its resolution and on the file compression. An uncompressed image with a resolution of 1,280 x 1,024 takes up 3.75 MB while an 800 x 600 image can be compressed to only100 KB.

A digital camera should have enough memory so that the images do not have to be downloaded to the computer too often. Thirty or forty images are usually sufficient for a whole day of shooting before downloading. Individual practice needs can vary, however.

To determine the amount of removable memory there is a need to add to the digital camera count,the number of pictures shot in an average day and double that number. Calculate the file dimension for each image at the quality required (this is not always the best possible quality). For example, if an average of 20 pictures per day and the digital camera saves the images in 200 KB files with acceptable quality, 8 MB memory is needed.

SPEED TO TRANSFER TO COMPUTER:

All images stored in the digital camera's memory are eventually transferred to a computer for archiving. The time needed to transfer the images depends on two factors: the size of the image files and the transfer speed (in KB / second). Since the file dimension is determined by the resolution and compression of the image, a reduction in size will have a negative impact on image quality. Therefore, transfer speed is the key variable.

There are two different ways to transfer the images from the camera to the computer:

1) Cable connection. Most digital cameras can be connected to a PC or Macintosh computer through a serial or parallel port. This kind of connection is extremely slow, however, and serial transfer is slower than parallel. Some cameras can use a SCSI port, which is much faster, but not available on all PCs.

2) Transfer from removable memory through a computer derive. This is probably the most convenient way to transfer the images to the computer.

If the digital camera uses compact flash cards, miniature cards, or SSFDCs, a PCMCIA drive is the method of choice. PCMCIA drives are built into all computers (both PC and Macintosh), but can also be mounted in any desktop PC. File transfer through a PCMCIA drive is extremely fast and easy.

If the camera uses a floppy disk for removable memory, the floppy drive of the computer can be used for file transfer. Floppy disk reading speeds are slow, however, and since each disk can hold only1.4 MB of data, only digital cameras that store files of limited size use them.

RECORD KEEPING

Orthodontic diagnostic records are taken for two purposes to document the starting point for treatment and to add to the information gathered on clinical examination. The records fall into three major categories:

1) Evaluation of the teeth and oral structures

2) Evaluation of the occlusion

3) Evaluation of facial and jaw proportions

Records for evaluation of the teeth and oral structures:

A major purpose of intraoral photographs, which should be obtained routinely for patients receiving complex orthodontic treatment, is to document the initial condition of the hard and soft tissues. Five standard intraoral photographs are suggested: right, center and left views with the teeth in occlusion, and maxillary and mandibular occlusal views. Maximum retraction of the cheeks and lips is needed. If there is a special soft tissue problem (e.g, no attached gingival in the lower anterior), an additional photograph of that area may be needed.

A panoramic intraoral radiograph is valuable for orthodontic evaluation at any age. The panoramic film has two significant advantages over a series of intraoral radiographs: it yields a broader view and thus is more likely to show any pathologic lesions and supernumerary or impacted teeth, and the radiation exposure is much lower. It also gives a view of the mandibular condyles, which can be helpful and as screening film to determine if other TMJ joint radiographs are needed.

The panoramic film should be supplemented with periapical and bitewing radiographs only when their greater details are required. In addition, for children and adolescents, periapical views of incisors are indicated if there is evidence or suspicion of root resorption. The principle is that periapical films to supplement the panoramic radiograph are ordered only if there is a specific indication of doing so.

Radiographs of the temporomandibular joint should be reserved for patients who have symptoms of dysfunction of that joint that might be related to internal joint pathology. In that case, CT or MRI scans are likely to be more useful than transcranial or lamina graphic TM joint films. Routine TM joint radiographs simply are not indicated for orthodontic patients.

Records for occlusal evaluation:

Evaluation of the occlusion requires impressions for dental casts or for digitization into computer memory and a record of the occlusion so that the casts or images can be related to each other.

Records for evaluation of facial properties:

For any orthodontic patient, facial and jaw proportions, not just dental occlusal relationship, must be evaluated. This can be done by a careful clinical evaluation of the patient's face, with a recording of positive findings, or by cephalometric radiographs if indicated.

CONCLUSION

Photography offers many advantages including rapid turn-around, checkable exposure accuracy, no ageing of photos, dust and scratch resistance, built in white balance, immediate viewing, no film or processing costs, inexpensive storage, easy retrieval, duplication & easy transmission around the world in seconds.

Dental world constitutes of microstructures that have to be recorded in a detailed manner, in order to perform patient education, documentation of records and treatment, illustration of lectures, publications and web connectivity of complicated cases.

Digital photography in orthodontics assumes importance for diagnostic and treatment planning procedures, as it is low cost and less technique sensitive when compared to cephalometry. Though photography cannot be an alternative for cephalometry in orthodontic diagnosis, the paradigm shift towards soft tissue has elevated the status of photography in treatment planning.

REFERENCES

- Kravets TP. Documents on the History of the Invention of Photography. Leningrad, Russia: Soviet Acad Sci; 1949.
- ANIC Milosevic: Basic principles for taking extraoral photographs.
- Laws R. The author's guide to controlling the photograph. J Prosthet Dent. 2001.
- Samavi S:A short guide to clinical digital photography in orthodontics.
- Goldstein MB. Digital photography in your dental practice. The why's, how's, and wherefore's. Dent Today.
- Christensen GJ. Important clinical uses for digital photography. J Am Dent Assoc. 2005.
- Pensler AV. Photography in the dental practice (I). Quintessence Int Dent Dig. 1983;14:745-751.
- Hutchinson I, Williams P. Digital cameras. Br J Orthod. 1999;26:326-331
- Eastman Kodak Company. Professional techniques in dental photography. In: Biomedical Photography: A Kodak Seminar in Print. 1st ed. Rochester, NY: Eastman Kodak Co.; 1976:17-37.
- Casaglia A, DeDominicis P, Arcuri L, Gargari M, OttriaL, Dental photography today, part 1: Basic concepts. ORAL & implantology.
- Wander P, Gordon P. Specific applications of dental photography. Br Dent J. 1987;162:393-403.
- Patel A: Clinical digital dental photography.CAD/CAM.
- Sandler J, Murray A. Digital photography in orthodontics. Journal of orthodontics.
- Sreesan NS, Purushothamam B, Rahul CS, Shafanath T, Fawaz V: Clinical photography in orthodontics.
- Sugawara Y, Saito K, Futaki M, Naruse M, Ono M, Hino R, Chiba Y: Evaluation of the optimal exposure settings for occlusal photograpy with digital cameras.

- Kumar M, MODI TG, Patel J, Sathwara N: Mastering camera systems in dentistry.
- Sharland MR: An update on digital photography for the general dental practitioner.
- Liu F, editor. Dental Digital photography for the general dental practitioner.
- Freeman M. The photographers studio manual.
- BengelW.Mastering digital dental photography..
- Abu Lghud JL: Newyork, Chicago, Losangeles, Americas Global Cities.
- Bengel W. Mastering digital dental photography.
- Snyder TC .Refine your dental photography, J Cosmet Dent 2013.
- Roldao E, P Arola AJ, Vilgarious M, Lavedrine B, Ramos AM. Unveiling the colors of cellulose nitrate black & white film based negatives in colonial photography.
- BengelW.Mastering digital dental photography.2006 March.
- Snow SR. Dental photography systems :required features for equipment selection .Compendium of continuity education in dentistry. 2005 May.
- Takashi K: The latest intraoral photographic techniques. Tokyo: Ishiyaku; 2007.
- Grey T. Color confidence .Alameda:Sybex; 2004.
- Zhang C, Zhang R, Ma X, Zhao Y. The choice and application of digital cameras in oral photography .Chin Aesthet Med .2003.
- PerttiPirttiniemi, Mastering digital dental photography (2006), *European Journal of Orthodontics*, Volume 28, Issue 6, December 2006, Page 624.
- Sharland MR. An update on digital photography for the general dental practitioner. *Dent Update*. 2008;35(6):398-404.
- Snow SR. Dental Photography Systems: Required Features for Equipment Selection. Compendium May 2005; Vol. 26.

www.ingramcontent.com/pod-product-compliance
Ingram Content Group UK Ltd.
Pitfield, Milton Keynes, MK11 3LW, UK
UKHW061023310726
14090UKWH00023B/49

9798897779970